MIRACLE BABES

God's Goodness in the Formation of Families

With Lindsey Racz, Jennifer Auxier, Karen Campbell, Laura Davis, Terah Hensley, Kelsey Grant, Kristina Lace, Shawna Landazuri, and Melissa Ridderbos

Foreword by: Sara Forhetz

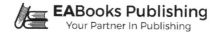

EABooks Publishing
Your Partner In Publishing

Cover design: Lauren Short and Matthew Racz

ISBN: 978-1-963611-36-6

Published by EA Books Publishing, a division of
Living Parables of Central Florida, Inc. a 501c3

EABooksPublishing.com

Table of Contents

DEDICATIONS

In Loving Memory of Janely Hope Landazuri whose 9 years on this earth touched more lives for Christ than we could imagine. In your legacy, may we remember to love fiercely, sing loudly, persevere suffering well, and never stop pointing others to Jesus.

And to the additional 20 miracles represented on these pages, may you never forget how deeply loved you are and how many desperate prayers were prayed just to know you: Solomon, Elijah, and Anna Kay; Caleb, Kate, and Allyson; Noel; Klaire, Kenlee, and Korinne; Andrew; Ben and Libby; Christiane, Kendy, and Kenda; Malakai, Brooke, Selah, and Ari.

FOREWORD

What a joy it is that you picked up this book. The stories of faith in the face of absolute heartbreak are both inspiring and challenging. After all, a faith that isn't challenged does not grow. I find it easy to walk by faith—fully trusting God when it's just Him and me at 5 a.m. on my living room couch. But when the rubber meets the road, when I am staring down a giant, a diagnosis, the unexpected loss of a loved one, another miscarriage, or some seemingly "pointless" heartache—that is where a faith that endures is developed.

It's in these darkest moments that we see His light shine, we feel His breath so closely, and truly rest peacefully in His presence.

The lessons learned on these pages are instructive for every reader, whether your personal journey includes infertility or not. Though your challenge might not be the same, reading about how these women learned to trust God deeper, hold on for longer than they ever thought possible—and still say, "It is well with my soul," can be an inspiring message for all of us.

I believe the Lord picked this book for you to encourage you to believe again, to trust an all-loving, all-Sovereign God with how your story unfolds.

But make no mistake, throughout the pages of Scripture, when many women who were identified as barren thought all hope was lost—many conceived. God brought forth life in Sarah, Hannah, Ruth, Elizabeth, the Shunamite woman, and beyond. Sarah gave birth to Isaac. Hannah gave birth to Samuel. Ruth gave birth to Obed. Elizabeth gave birth to John the Baptizer, who was the forerunner to the most important miraculous conception of all—Jesus.

And while we learn much from the children they all bore, we learn equally, and as valuable, lessons from their mommas' journeys, too. While your journey is unique, you are certainly not alone. Someone, somewhere, has walked a similar path. Jesus sees you. He weeps with you. And His joy comes in the morning. In the waiting, you will find His strength perfected in you. You will lack no good thing in Him.

Each woman mentioned above spent a considerable amount of time struggling with her barrenness. Ultimately, she conceived when God knew the appointed time had come. Not one day, or one decade too soon, and not one moment too late.

What if, at this time next year, you were holding the hand of your own child? What if you had him or her naturally? What if you adopted, as is encouraged in Scripture? ("Religion that God our Father accepts as pure and faultless is this: to look after orphans and widows in their distress and to keep oneself from being polluted by the world." James 1:27) What if your "yes" to God kept a child of God from being polluted in this current culture? What if a phone call comes from a friend or relative, or from a family in your church or workplace—to raise a child who needs a home? What if with high hopes, high faith, and an unrelenting "Yes, Lord, be it unto me as you have said," (Luke 1:38) you open yourself up to God-sized dreams and possibilities?

Perhaps your "for such a time as this" moment is just around the corner. Maybe our lives are not entirely about us, but about the multitudes around us who are gleaning from our faith, courage, and perseverance. From the wisdom and persistence in our faith we only learn by walking through this season.

Our God is for you, not against you. Nothing that is impossible for man is impossible for God. While we wait on His perfect timing, we must keep our faith that He is working together a plan for our good. While not every story ended up looking the way these women had originally hoped it would, what God gave them was even more beautiful than they had dreamed. "For now we see through a glass, darkly;

but then face to face: now I know in part; but then shall I know even as also I am fully known" (1 Corinthians 13:12).

We're not always granted understanding this side of Heaven. But in Christ, we are granted the faith that is God-given, to believe "His ways are higher, and His thoughts are higher, and He is accomplishing what He intends to accomplish" (Isaiah 55). Only in a relationship with Jesus can His children, every time, look and say, "it is good." My faith, my trust, my resolve, my commitment to an all-powerful God has grown just reading how the Lord worked out so many twist-and-turn details in the lives of the families represented on these pages.

By any worldly standard, no one would say my story was "good" either. But once I met this God—the only one who can take all things and work them together for His glory and my good (Romans 8:28), can I say this—God has brought beauty from my ashes. He has restored to me the years the locust has stolen (Joel 2:25). And He's used every bit of heartache to draw others to Himself out of my testimony. I trust Him deeper because of the difficulties I have faced.

My prayer is that your challenges will draw you close to Him; may the way you face your struggles lead others to believe in Him. May the chapters that lie ahead refine you. But remember, your story is still being written—and so are theirs. It's not over until the coming of the Son of Man. And even then, it's only just beginning.

GOD, FAMILIES, AND MIRACLES
By Lindsey Racz

I've heard it said that a true miracle involves intervention from the divine, resulting in an extraordinary event that otherwise would not be possible in the human world. I wonder what brought you to these pages. Perhaps you know one of the Miracle Babe authors. Perhaps you picked up this book on a whim. Or perhaps, just maybe, you're in need of a miracle of your own. It doesn't matter how you got here, but it does matter that you are here. You belong here on these pages with us. As you read about our miracles, some stories may not meet your expectation of a "miracle"— happily stringing along details until no pain is left. They won't sound this way because on this earth, we will experience suffering . . .

Infertility. A child with special needs. Adoption.

These words and phrases are laced with pain and heartache. But look closer. Within our stories lie the deep miracle of human life. With all of our heartaches, despair, unmet longings, and unspoken dreams, God is doing something bigger. He is working on miracles.

God first spoke to me about *Miracle Babes* in December of 2022. I was a new business owner running a rapidly growing women's mental health clinic in Springfield, Missouri and struggling to keep my head above water. Between seeing clients, learning how to run a business, having supervisees, purchasing a new building for our clinic, serving in my church's children's ministry, and family life, the demands on my time were endless. I was near burnout, if not wallowing in it, when I attended a women's conference with my new neighbor.

Flourish was the theme of the conference; it was a typical women's ministry event with breakout sessions, worship, and lots of studying God's Word. I needed it. And I needed more. I became enthralled with a faithful woman who taught one of the breakout sessions about discipleship.

Sally Herman was a retired nurse who had raised a family of her own and was now actively serving in her church, discipling countless women how to walk closer to Christ. Sally also happened to be my neighbor's mother-in-law. After the conference, I sidled up to my neighbor and asked how her mother-in-law was so vibrant in her faith after years of serving. Wasn't she tired? My neighbor smiled and, soon after, she brought me a pamphlet that Sally had written on the topic of retreating with God.

I once heard about people who take retreats with God. In my college years when I sat under the ministry of on-fire leaders, they spoke of their "getaways" with the Lord. Some would go to remote campgrounds. Others retreated to their room for a weekend, and some even visited monasteries. Somehow over the years, I had not taken time to squeeze in a retreat with God, but I desperately wanted to be vibrant like these people. After 20 years of living as a sold-out follower of Christ, I was tired. Life had been hard, expectations had gone unmet, and some of my dreams had died. Although there were many blessings all around me, I knew in the moments of devouring Sally Herman's pamphlet about a God-retreat, that it was time for me to get alone with the One who could restore my soul.

I happen to live in a small college town. We have one large state university, one private university, and a large technical college all within our city boundary. During the summer and winter breaks when students go home to their families, our traffic gets quite a bit lighter. There's space to breathe.

As I began to dream about taking a retreat alone, a friend of mine who has rental properties near campus came to mind. Perhaps one of her lovely homes would be available in early December. A few texts later, my first ever retreat alone with God was set. I would stay at Trish's immaculate and Pinterest-style historic home for a full weekend with the sole purpose of reconnecting my soul to the God of the universe. Oh, how I was desperate to shut out the noise of the world and be alone with Him.

I went into my retreat with no expectations other than some peace and quiet. I was hungry to hear from God but wasn't sure I would. I was seeking His wisdom specifically about business decisions that were looming. Armed with the journals I had kept my entire adult life, a bible, and a fresh new journal, I entered the weekend unsure how God would direct me.

During those two days I prayed a lot, read through my old journals, and danced to worship music on the charming, creaky wooden floors. Reading through the journals was insightful and one particular season of journaling kept calling me back. One journal, written between 2015-2018, contained the tale of our behind-the-scenes battle with infertility, receiving a miracle pregnancy, and then getting the news that this new baby I was carrying was actually very sick. To be honest, I must have pushed those painful years away, but in the quiet of the retreat as I read my own story, the wound stung fresh. I remembered the heartache as if it were just happening instead of being five years in the rear-view mirror.

Somewhere on the second day of that retreat, my pen started writing. Yes, I was holding it, but I didn't come up with the words it was scribbling down almost faster than my hand could keep up. The words read:

MIRACLE BABES: Tales of God's Goodness in the Formation of Families

And then came a list of multiple women's names, and finally, one last sentence: "All proceeds are to go to the Pregnancy Care Center."

The process of writing down these details took less than five minutes, and yet when I reread those words, I knew I had just received direct marching orders from a God who indeed came to meet with me at our retreat. I tucked the journal away, finished my retreat with time in His word, and went back to the hustle and bustle of everyday life.

December 11th was a Monday. We were knee deep in the details of purchasing a new clinic for our mental health practice that would need a complete remodel, if not rehabilitation. I was also in Christmas preparation mode with our family. The days moved quickly, and it would have been easy to forget about the directive God gave in the quiet moments alone with Him just days earlier. It would have been easier to say "no thank you" to this monumental task . . . except that the Holy Spirit wouldn't let me do that. Truly, I did argue a bit. "God, I'm so busy. I don't even personally know some of these women whose names you've given me! Is there someone else who might be better at heading up this collaboration? Please? Also, God, I know nothing about the Pregnancy Care Center. They appear to do good work that honors you, but I don't know about their internal structure and value systems. I don't know about their work culture. I've never even been there!"

Then go find out.

This was the still small voice, the nudge that pushed back on my spirit. Like a child who endlessly rattles excuses and the parent who calmly yet firmly replies, "I've already given you an answer", the conversation went on for several days. The choice lay before me. I could be obedient and walk in the calling I felt had been entrusted to me, or I could pretend I had made it all up and continue with my all-consuming work in the mental health field. After all, we were running a Christian counseling clinic and already doing Kingdom work. What more could the Lord ask of me? Thankfully, my history with the Lord runs deep and rich; He's given me plenty of examples of what happens when I choose my own way over His. Spoiler alert: it never ends well.

Obedience meant my next step was to reach out to our town's pregnancy care center and schedule a tour so I could learn more about their mission, values, and culture. The day of our tour, the woman I had been corresponding with via email must have been out, because the woman who actually led me through the clinic was the Executive Director herself: Lisa McIntire. Lisa is one of those women who exudes love, confidence, and depth. She guided me down every hall on every floor, showing me training and counseling rooms, introducing me to staff and volunteers, all the while sharing the nonprofit's vision for families. 417 PCC, as it's known locally, offers services for planned and unplanned pregnancies. They support mothers and fathers with services that are free because they are covered by donors in our community and beyond. Many pregnant teens have walked through their doors, seen and heard a tiny heartbeat on a screen, and chosen life. Many adoptions have been initiated within the walls of the clinic. Many teenage and adult men have grown in their confidence to show up as dads and have learned what it means to be a father.

Father. Now that's a word that's close to God's heart. God is the ultimate Father and we are the family knit into His heart. We are His dream. In the same way you've perhaps dreamt of having a family of your own, of being a mom, of holding a baby tightly to your chest, God's heart dreamt also of us. You see, He is a triune God. Scripture tells us that God exists as Father, Son, and the Holy Spirit. This means that relationships and fellowship are woven into His very nature. He longed to grow His family, to multiply His love; His dream became reality when, miracle of miracles, He made us.

Gotquestions.org continues this discussion:

> The concept of family is extremely important in the Bible, both in a physical sense and in a theological sense. The concept of family was introduced in the very beginning, as we

see in Genesis 1:28, "God blessed them and said to them, 'Be fruitful and increase in number; fill the earth and subdue it. Rule over the fish of the sea and the birds of the air and over every living creature that moves on the ground.'" God's plan for creation was for men and women to marry and have children. A man and a woman would form a "one-flesh" union through marriage (Genesis 2:24), and they with their children become a family, the essential building block of human society. (GotQuestions.org, 2010)

Families are part of God's grand design. They gift us depth and understanding about the world. They teach us about God's parental, sacrificial love for us and provide caring and stable environments for children to learn about God's protective love. Safety. Belonging. Fullness. A family, in its truest form, is a picture of heaven.

But families need not be narrowly defined and left to only those traditional standards. Regardless of our marital or parental status, we are already part of a family. If we believe in Christ and the sacrifice He made, we are adopted into God's glorious family. We already belong! Longing for a family is a natural reflection of being created in God's image. His dreams are written on our hearts; yet let us pause and acknowledge that He has already fulfilled our desire to be held, safe, and part of something bigger than ourselves.

We live in a fallen world where no family is left untouched by conflict and dysfunction. No one knows this better than those of us who work as therapists. Our job is to "pull the curtain back" in our client's lives, so to speak. We see what's behind the perfect family photo on social media into the darkness and heartache that exists between humans when sin enters the picture. There is no pain that can reach the depths of the human soul like the pain of a crumbling family. When families come apart because of death, infertility, illness, divorce, addiction, or any other means of loss, the human heart breaks.

The story of life often doesn't go as we plan. The plot twists seem unsavory. The outcomes are not what we would have chosen. Or are they? As powerfully profound author and speaker Katherine Wolf is known for saying, "Perhaps some detours aren't detours at all. Perhaps they are actually the path."

So, what about your path? Have you always longed for a family? Have you hoped against hope for your family to be whole? Have you pleaded with God for healing? Are you struggling with infertility? A new diagnosis for your child? Does your heart's cry to be a parent feel like an open wound as the doctor delivers the news that you'll never have children? That your baby is sick? Have you lost a child?

Dearest reader, God is still working. My deepest prayer is that you'll find yourself in our stories as the Creator of life continues to write yours. If your heart needs mending, be encouraged. He *is* love and human hearts are put back together by love. The Lord cares deeply about knitting families together—even and especially through shattered dreams—He works, weaves, and breathes life. Look up; miracles happen on ordinary days.

REFERENCES

GotQuestions.org. (2010, March 29). *Home.* https://www.gotquestions.org/Bible-family.html

CHAPTER ONE

IN THE MIDST

By Melissa Ridderbos

I always assumed I'd have children. Maybe two or three. I'd find a great husband, buy that house with the white picket fence, get a dog, and have some babies. Easy breezy, right? Things had always gone pretty well for me in life, so why would I assume any differently in this case? Oh, how young and naive I was. Can't we all say that when we look back on our younger selves, though? It's not that we shouldn't dream big or assume good things for our lives, but rather, we need to be equipped for when things don't go according to plan. The track of our lives can be filled with some pretty big hurdles, and I've encountered quite a few.

THE FIRST HURDLE WAS FINDING A HUSBAND.

I got married much later in life than most of my friends, much to my chagrin. I had been in quite a few relationships over the years, but I always felt like something was missing, not realizing at the time that thing was God. I was a bit of a lost soul with little direction. After college, I moved back in with my parents to my childhood home in Maryland and began working as a receptionist at a small marketing company. Shortly after, my boyfriend at the time decided to move to Missouri for grad school. I did not have a strong career focus, and a big move sounded fun, so at the wise old age of 22 I decided to move halfway across the country from Maryland to Missouri (sorry Mom and Dad!). I was seeking in every aspect of my life during that season; I was seeking change, adventure, purpose, and meaning. When my relationship ended, even though my entire family was back in Maryland, for some reason I felt compelled to stay in Missouri. I had found a job I loved at a wonderful, small, family-run company and was really enjoying my new friends and adventures living on my own.

ENTER GOD.

There was something special about the company I was working for in Missouri. The people were all so kind and friendly, there were Bible verses on the walls all around the office, and they even held optional Bible studies during lunch breaks. I was not a Christian at that point in my life, so you can imagine how strange this all felt to me at first. Growing up, my family did not go to church or talk about God much. We celebrated Christmas and had a little nativity set I loved playing with as a kid, but I never understood the true meaning behind it all. When I was very young, I remember being distraught over big life topics that I couldn't understand, like the fact that humans experience death, and what happens after we die. I was left questioning with no answers to satisfy me. Despite having a wonderful childhood and a loving family, I struggled with some anxiety and insecurities as I got older. I found my self-worth from things like people's approval of me and my physical looks. Regarding religion, I considered myself agnostic and was rather critical in my heart towards people who talked about Jesus or believed the Bible was true. I would *never* have guessed that years later I would end up becoming one of them!

Over the years working for this company, God truly changed me. I began asking questions about the Bible and Jesus, attending church occasionally, doing lots of research, and experiencing God in ways I never had before. I was unsure what I believed at that point, but I was open, asking, and seeking (Matthew 7:7).

One of my favorite memories from this time was when I was going through another breakup with yet another boyfriend. One of my new Christian friends offered to pray for me while we were sitting in her car after lunch one day, so I said, "Aww, sure, that's nice of you." I thought that was just a nice thing for her to say, like many people casually say, "I'm praying for you." But then she proceeded to close her eyes and actually pray *out loud* for me right then and there, talking to God so intimately and genuinely. It honestly felt very strange and a little uncomfortable. No one had ever done that for me before. And you know what? I loved it! I felt this amazing presence in the car with us, like I was truly loved and known. That was the first of many times people prayed out loud with me, and to this day, there is just something so powerful to it. Hello, Holy Spirit!

ENTER TIM.

Would you believe that after seven years of working at this company and many seasons of dating and singleness, they hired a man who would eventually become my husband? There was an obvious spark between us right from the beginning, but Tim and I were just friends for a while–a long while–like, a whole *year* to be exact (not that anyone was counting). Tim was a Christian who took his faith very seriously and understandably desired to have a wife with the same beliefs. He did not disclose that to me at the time, however, because he wanted me to decide for myself what I believed, and not just change my beliefs for him. He later told me he had been praying with his friends, and many of our coworkers, that I would come to know the Lord someday. He cared deeply about me and only wanted the best for me, even if it meant having patience on his part and waiting to see what God would do. To this day, I still admire how he never pushed his beliefs on me, rather he quietly and humbly lived out his faith in front of me. Tim was someone I deeply respected and trusted and became one of my closest friends. He was always there for me and helped me wrestle through so many hard questions I had about life, the Bible, and Jesus.

ENTER FAITH.

One thing the company I worked for did really well was showing me how to put faith into action. They did not simply *post* bible verses on the walls; they strived to put those verses into practice. For example, they started a charity organization with the heart to help children in orphanages, and they offered employees the opportunity to go with this organization on mission trips to Haiti. I had never done anything like that before, and as our plane descended over the tent-filled landscape, it didn't take long to realize I had been living in a bubble my whole life. My first trip to Haiti took me way out of my comfort zone and taught me so many things. One of the biggest lessons was seeing that God is everywhere and that oftentimes people who have far less physically can have so much more spiritually. We attended a small, dilapidated church one day that did not even have a roof, and I witnessed the most joyful, beautiful people, singing out to God! We also visited orphanages and played with children living in the saddest circumstances, yet somehow they taught me about finding joy in the simple things. Coming back to America was very hard. I felt extremely guilty for my privileged life, but I turned my guilt into gratitude, and God used the experience to make me a better person.

When we got back to the states, I contemplated everything I had experienced and finally came to a point where I could not deny that God is real! After years of seeking, God softened my heart and opened my eyes to see my own sin and my need for a Savior. I realized I had been separated from God, but he longed to have a relationship with me. I realized the word "sinner" is not just for murderers; we all have sin in our hearts and must fight against it our entire lives. I realized the Bible is not just a book of stories; it is actual history that is relevant to how we live our lives today. It teaches us who Jesus is and about God's ultimate plan of redemption. I accepted God's free gift of salvation by declaring that Jesus is Lord, and by believing in my heart that He died to pay the penalty for my sins.

Shortly after becoming a Christian, and I mean *very* shortly, Tim asked me if he could "pursue a relationship" with me (what a gentleman!). We were engaged one year later and married six months after that, when I was 31 years old. What a gift God gave me in Tim. I can now look back, over all the heartbreaks and frustrations, and see how God's hand was in all the details of bringing us together. More importantly I see that God wanted me to pursue a relationship with *Him* before any human man. After that, the husband part fell right into place in God's perfect timing.

THE SECOND HURDLE WAS HAVING A BABY.

Before we got engaged, Tim and I had many conversations about what we wanted in life, one thing being our shared desire to have children. When we first got married, we made our neat and tidy plans to enjoy some kid-free time for a while, to focus on each other, travel, and ultimately enjoy being DINKS (Dual Income No Kids, as we jokingly referred to that time period). We adopted a sweet puppy as a practice child and boy did she prove to be great practice! About a year later, when I was 33 years old, we both felt that tug on our hearts that we wanted to have a baby. That is when things got hard.

Month after month, pee stick after pee stick, one ovulation tracking test after another, and no baby. *When do you start worrying if something is wrong? How long is too long? Am I too old? Is something wrong with me? With Tim? Why isn't this working, God? Everyone I know has kids! They make it look so easy!* The phone would ring and it would be another friend telling me her exciting news . . . she was pregnant . . . again. I felt truly happy for each friend, but when I hung up the phone, I would begin sobbing. Oh, how I longed to experience the magic of pregnancy, the unique experience of breastfeeding, the bond between a mother and her child. It was devastating. I couldn't handle going to another baby shower or another gender reveal party. It was all around me, all the time. I cried in Tim's arms more times than I can count and pleaded with God, *Why God? When is it going to be MY turn?*

THEN THE SEASON OF PEOPLE'S WELL-INTENTIONED ADVICE.

"Aww, you guys just need to relax."

"Try not to stress; stress is so hard on the body."

"Try this."

"Try that."

"It will happen when you stop trying so hard."

But in our minds, we were not trying any harder than anyone else. It just wasn't happening. So we began investigating why. Tim visited his doctor and got a clean bill of health. We then went to a doctor who specialized in women's health issues. During an investigative procedure, he discovered that both of my fallopian tubes were blocked, I had a cyst on one of my ovaries, and I had stage 3 endometriosis. All of these things affect fertility, but the doctor said he could help us and gave us a lot of hope. I had surgery to open my fallopian tubes, remove the cyst and excise all of the endometriosis, and shortly after healing, we continued trying to get pregnant. It felt so good to have some answers and a renewed hope! But a full year later, there was still no baby. *Why God?* We were getting very discouraged.

Our next step was to consider in vitro fertilization (IVF). We knew a few friends who had success with this method, but let me tell you, it did not settle well with me at first. As a Christian, I couldn't help but wonder what God thinks of IVF. *Does doing IVF mean we are not trusting God anymore, like we are taking it into our own hands? Does God approve of IVF? What would happen to any leftover embryos? Do I really want to put my body through all of the invasive procedures and medications?* I had so many questions and so many worries. I did not want to play God, rather, I wanted God to make these big decisions for us. Tim was feeling many of the same things, however, he ultimately had more peace about IVF than I did. We sought advice and prayer from our pastor, friends, and family, and we prayed over the decision for a long time. We even specifically prayed, "Lord, if we do IVF, please make it so that there aren't any leftover embryos." After a lot of research and prayer, we finally came to the conclusion that God is pro-life, and He loves to make families. He created science and gave humans the ability and creativity to invent things like IVF to aid in our brokenness. With this new mindset, I remember sitting on Tim's lap one night and saying to him, "If you really want to do this and truly feel God is leading us to try IVF, I will try it." We both cried happy tears. It was a big sacrifice for me, but we are called in marriage to make sacrifices and ultimately God gave me so much peace about it. This was a sweet, special moment in our marriage that God used to bring us closer to Him and to each other.

IVF was an adventure to say the least; I never imagined my husband would be giving me injections in my rear! It was hard on my body, very time consuming, and very expensive, but with God's help I felt strong and empowered and hopeful through the whole process. I truly believed IVF was going to be our answer . . . sadly, it was not. We had two viable embryos, but after having both implanted inside my uterus, and after all the money, and all the medications and all the anticipation, we received the news by phone one day that our IVF had failed. *Why God?* Our renewed hope had once again ended in disappointment.

While processing our emotions, we were forced to face the fact that we may never have biological children. It would have been easy to be angry with God at that point, but we tried our best to trust God's timing and plan for our lives (Jeremiah 29:11). Scripture is full of encouragement and promises from God, so we clung to those with all our strength. My faith was growing a lot during that time, and I remember finally coming to a place where I truly felt peace if we never had kids. "Your will be done," I prayed to God one day, and I truly meant it. We knew God loved us and the Bible tells us that He works all things together for good for those who love Him (Romans 8:28), so we trusted that His plan, no matter what it was, was good. It was not easy to get to this place of peace. It was a long, hard journey with lots of tears, but ultimately every good and perfect gift is from above (James 1:17), and God is the one in control. God gave us peace that surpasses understanding and covered us with His love throughout the entire IVF process. Going through this part of our journey made us stronger as individuals and as a couple, and I can see now how God was involved in all the details, even our concern about what we would do if we had leftover embryos. Remember how we prayed to have no leftover embryos? God was so kind to answer that prayer.

Additionally, throughout our IVF journey, God was so good to introduce us to some wonderful people we may have never met otherwise. In fact, would you believe I met the lead author of this very book, Lindsey Racz, while sitting in the waiting room of the IVF clinic one day? We became fast friends, sharing our similar stories, and Lindsey went on to become an incredible support to me throughout our whole infertility journey. I praise God for bringing her into my life and for all the ways she has inspired me and helped me become a stronger woman.

OKAY, BACK TO BABIES.

Even though God blessed us so much through our IVF journey, we still did not have a baby, the true desire of our hearts (Psalm 37:4). One day we saw an ad that a local church was hosting an event to educate people about foster care and adoption, so we decided to attend. At one point during the presentation, Tim and I looked over at each other and we were both ugly crying; like, entire face wet, mascara-running-down-cheeks type of crying. We were so moved by the touching, wonderful stories of how God created these families through foster care and adoption. It was so inspiring. We knew for sure we were not done building our family. Shortly after, we visited an adoption agency to learn more and began the process of filling out an application to become foster parents. At the same time, there was still a part of us that deeply desired to have a biological child, so we also decided to begin the process of trying IVF again. What happened next still gives me chills. Right before we turned in our foster care paperwork, and right before we signed the big deposit check for our second round of IVF, God gave us the surprise of a lifetime!

It was December, and Christmas was approaching, my favorite time of the year. God had blessed us in so many ways like great friendships, a wonderful church, lovely neighbors, and financial stability. My period was late again, but by this time we had stopped counting days or getting excited as my periods had been late many times over the last few years.

For some reason, this time, I decided to take a pregnancy test while Tim was still at work. Within seconds, the test showed . . . POSITIVE! *What? Oh my goodness could this actually be true?* I was shaking with nerves and excitement. I knew I wouldn't be able to hide my excitement from Tim when he got home that night, so I made a plan to surprise him right away.

Since it was almost Christmas we had stockings hanging on our mantle, so I hid the pregnancy test in Tim's stocking. Tim called and said he had some errands to run after work, but I insisted he come home right away (not suspicious at all). When he walked in the house, I told him I had an early Christmas gift for him and to go look in his stocking.

The look on his face was priceless! I found an old journal entry I wrote right after we found out this news that sums up how we were both feeling:

> *Dear Lord, can this be true? A positive pregnancy test after three and a half years of trying, a failed IVF, and after we*

ALMOST paid for another round of IVF with a different doctor? Lord, if this is true, thank you so much for this miracle! Thank you for giving us peace while we waited on your perfect timing. Please, Lord, please help this to be true and help the baby to be healthy and happy and know you as soon as possible. We know you already know him/her as you are the one who creates life and knits them together in my womb. Help me to take good care of myself and have a healthy happy pregnancy, Lord. Help us to lean on you through everything! Please help this to be true Lord, please! What a perfect Christmas gift from you at the same time as you came down to earth over 2000 years ago to save the world from its sins! Yes Lord, you are a God of miracles!! Nothing and I mean nothing is impossible with you. God, thank you so much for this healthy pregnancy inside of me. My dream come true, my wish, my prayer. A true gift from you, Lord. Help us to have peace and trust you in all of this Lord. In your holy name, Amen.

Nine months later, God blessed us with a perfectly amazing baby girl. What a *miracle babe* our Noel is to us. We are so incredibly in love with her and blessed by her life. Life sure was different after that, but life was good.

MORE HURDLES.

Our baby story was not over. Shortly after Noel turned two years old, we were shocked to find out I was pregnant again! We announced it very quickly to both of our families as we could not hide our excitement. I felt very sick the entire first month, which was the same for my first pregnancy, so we had no reason to believe that anything would go wrong. Nothing could have prepared us for what happened next. We went in for our first routine ultrasound appointment, and as the technician got more and more quiet, we knew something was wrong. Finally the doctor came in and told us she was so sorry but they could not find a heartbeat. We were devastated. I even went and got a second opinion because my mind refused to believe it. How could I have been so sick, so miserable, for weeks, but now this? I went in for a D&C procedure a week later, and we once again experienced the pain of loss and disappointment. *Why God?* This was the beginning of one of the hardest years of our marriage.

A few months after our miscarriage, I received another surprise of a lifetime . . . breast cancer. *Me? Seriously? They must have read the results wrong or mixed up my paperwork.* Cancer did not run in my family. I was young and healthy and would never have imagined something like this would happen to me. This is when I got better at not asking "Why God?" anymore and stopped leaning on my own understanding (Proverbs 3:5). I learned to lean hard on my faith, and with God's help, face things one day at a time. Things moved very quickly after that; paperwork, doctors' appointments, scans, and more doctors' appointments. My head was spinning. I went in to get a port implanted into my chest and got started on chemotherapy right away. Five months later I had a double mastectomy, followed by another full year of a different type of chemo. Fighting cancer was a brutal and difficult journey, but as strange as it may sound, God blessed me during those two years and made me feel extra loved. I found another journal entry I wrote during my cancer journey that speaks to this:

> *Somehow in the midst of all this pain and discomfort, you are making me feel so loved, Lord. Everything that once felt mundane or uninspiring, is so much more inspiring now. When you've experienced the agony of true pain and suffering, a simple evening pain free, sitting outside with no bugs and a break from this horrible heat we've been having, feels like heaven! My 3-year-old daughter telling me I am beautiful and telling me she loves me (and not even noticing my baldness*

for a split second), is just the kindest thing God could do. I even take my wig off right in front of her and she doesn't say a word . . . kids at that age don't notice or judge appearances. How refreshing!! A new friendship with neighbors (2 of which are dogs, lol . . . twin yellow labs to be exact) brings such joy to Noel's life, and to mine too. Noel runs down to our shared fence every single day to "talk" to Bonnie and Bailey! God is so good. A surprise visit from a friend and spiritual mentor of mine brought me to tears the other night. She prayed out loud over me and made me feel so known and loved. A sweet elderly lady working at the Panera drive through the other day looked directly and deep into my eyes (through our masks and through my silly wig which she was unaware was covering a bald head from cancer), and as she passed me my food she said, very intentionally with a big smile, "God bless you, Melissa, I hope you have a beautiful day!" Yep, I drove away and bawled my eyes out. I felt like Jesus was speaking to me through her. It was overwhelming in a spiritual sense I can't describe. Noel is going to a Mother's Day Out program once a week, and the teachers and directors are the kindest, Godly women, TWO of whom went through breast cancer too! I know she will be so loved there. I could go on and on about how present God feels in my life lately. Some people may think, what's the big deal, she's just had a lucky streak lately. But I know it's not luck. God is providing and helping me get through this crazy season of my life. And don't get me wrong, things have been very hard at times, but I want others to know, if they are going through a hard time or find themselves very stressed or lacking joy, to cast their cares to the Lord. Call to Him. Cry out to Him. Find rest. He loves us and wants to help us. He created us in our mother's womb and knows every detail of our being and He longs for an intimate personal relationship with us.

THEN CAME OUR MOST RECENT HURDLE.

And it was a doozy. At one of our oncology appointments, well into my cancer treatments, we were talking with my doctor about whether or not we could try to have kids again. She gave us a look that said it all. Due to the damaging effects of chemo on my ovaries and the need to take estrogen blocking medications for five to ten years, it was highly advised not to get pregnant, and most likely not even possible. Even if my ovaries were not too damaged from the chemo and miraculously woke back up, I would have to stop all of my medications, and even if a miracle pregnancy occurred, it would flood my body with estrogen (which is one of the things that fed the cancer cells). It would be an extremely high risk for both the baby and me, so basically "No." Realizing this news, we felt heartache once again. It was already hard enough to go through the miscarriage a few months earlier, then to suffer through all the hardships of breast cancer treatments, major surgery, and the physical changes to my body as a result of those treatments, but then to be told we would never be able to have kids again . . . it still brings tears to my eyes. Honestly, I think I am still in denial. I feel too young to not be able to have another baby, and my mind refuses to accept this is true most days. Noel is just getting to the age where she realizes she is the only one of her friends without a sibling, and she begs us for a baby sister many days. Life can be so hard and confusing. I know earlier in this story I wrote that God gave us so much peace at various points in our journey, but for some reason, Tim and I do not feel peace about this . . . yet. We are anxious to see what God does next.

**LET US RUN WITH PERSEVERANCE THE RACE
MARKED OUT FOR US.**

In life we will experience both joy and sorrow, sometimes simultaneously. The Bible tells us to reflect on our blessings and to think about good things (Philippians 4:4-9). Focusing on the good in our lives and practicing gratitude and contentment has helped us tremendously through these hurdles. While I am still grieving losses, I am very happy to say that I am cancer-free and loving being a mother to our miracle babe! Somehow in the midst of all these trials, God brought blessings. It's what He does. The creator of this universe is a loving heavenly Father, who comforts us in our pain and is faithful to meet all of our needs. He will use our trials to bring us closer to Him, to help us refocus on what is most important in life, and to help others going through similar trials. Most importantly, God's Word provides *hope* for the future. If you are in the midst of pain or sorrow, I pray you will seek God with all your heart and allow Him to be your fortress through it all.

SCRIPTURES REFERENCED

Jeremiah 29:11—For I know the plans I have for you, declares the Lord, plans to prosper you and not to harm you, plans to give you a hope and a future.

Romans 8:28—And we know that God causes everything to work together for the good of those who love God and are called according to his purpose for them.

James 1:17—Whatever is good and perfect is a gift coming down to us from God our Father, who created all the lights in the heavens. He never changes or casts a shifting shadow.

Psalm 37:4—Delight yourself in the Lord, and he will give you the desires of your heart.

Proverbs 3:5—Trust in the Lord with all your heart, and do not lean on your own understanding.

Philippians 4:4-9—Rejoice in the Lord always. I will say it again: Rejoice! Let your gentleness be evident to all. The Lord is near. Do not be anxious about anything, but in every situation, by prayer and petition, with thanksgiving, present your requests to God. And the peace of God, which transcends all understanding, will guard your hearts and your minds in Christ Jesus. Finally, brothers and sisters, whatever is true, whatever is noble, whatever is right, whatever is pure, whatever is lovely, whatever is admirable, if anything is excellent or praiseworthy, think about such things. Whatever you have learned or received or heard from me, or seen in me, put it into practice. And the God of peace will be with you.

Hebrews 12:1-2—Therefore, since we are surrounded by such a great cloud of witnesses, let us throw off everything that hinders and the sin that so easily entangles. And let us run with perseverance the race marked out for us, fixing our eyes on Jesus, the pioneer and perfecter of faith.

CHAPTER TWO

TEACH ME, LORD, TO WAIT

By Jen Auxier

I stared at the computer screen. There were nearly two dozen tabs open at the top of my browser about "starting the adoption process." We were 15 minutes into this whole adoption thing, and I was already feeling overwhelmed. My husband, David, had his laptop open doing the same Google searches.

"Where do we even start?" he asked me.

"I have no idea." I responded.

From a young age, I knew getting pregnant would be a difficult process for me. I was diagnosed with PCOS in my twenties and my body never quite figured out the whole reproductive cycle. We tried fertility treatments for a short time, but I hated the mood swings, constant monitoring of my cycle, and having to go to the doctor for bi-weekly blood draws. So after a few "failed" months of trying to get pregnant, it was an easy decision for us to pursue adoption. We had talked about adopting a child on one of our first dates. My grandfather had been the director of an adoption agency and David had vivid memories of church services that led him to believe God was calling him to be an adoptive parent. We knew at some point adoption would be part of our story, but we planned to have our own biological children first.

During the first year of our marriage, we lived in a suburb of Kansas City, Missouri. I worked as a middle school teacher, and David was working as a high school Bible teacher at a private school but pursuing a career as a Senior Pastor. We fully believed that God had called him to be a pastor, so he was sending resumes all over as we continued to pray for God's direction. A year into our marriage, God led my husband to take a new job as the senior pastor of a small church in rural southern Illinois. This meant we needed to move to another state. I did not want to move. I had grown up and put down roots in the same town and I was happy with my house, my career, and my social life. Kansas City was home, but God was clearly calling us away, so I begrudgingly uprooted and when God said go, I went.

This turned out to be one of God's little graces throughout the process. David had a family friend, Regina, who was a social worker for the Illinois Baptist Children's Home, so we put the Google searches behind us and contacted her to start the adoption process. We lived an hour from her office, which was nothing considering that we also lived 40 minutes from a discount store and 75 minutes from the nearest coffee place! It truly was a rural town. We were able to meet with Regina and she began to guide us through the daunting process.

Regina gave us the paperwork needed to start our home study. The packet was nearly two inches thick with pages and pages of tasks. We needed 10 letters of recommendations, updated physicals, three different types of background checks, and we had to write multiple essays about our family, child rearing philosophies, and personal histories. My goal was to complete the home study in three months, but moving to a new state, starting a new job, and getting settled into a new church meant that completing the package took seven months. In the grand scheme of things, seven months is not a long time, but when your heart is set on holding a new baby, it feels like eternity.

In the meantime, I had to come to terms with my infertility. My social media feed was filled with birth announcements and the TV was filled with baby ads. Every time I went shopping, all I could see was the adorable baby section. I had many nights of feeling sorry for myself when I would cry and question God's plan. All I wanted was to be a mom, but that dream seemed unattainable. The questions poured out. *Why did it have to be so hard? Why did I have to go through this? Why did I have to provide my last three years of tax returns, go through 40+ hours of training, have a health physical, background check, and provide a letter from my employer to have a baby while that random lady at the grocery store had four kids she couldn't keep track of?* I was angry. In my heart, I knew God was good, but in my mind, I thought He was withholding good from us.

I did the only thing I knew to do; turn to the Bible. Hannah's story became my lifeline and I read the account in First Samuel over and over. I felt Hannah's humiliation as her husband's second wife provoked her for not having a child. I knew her anguish as she begged God for a son. I understood the tension between wanting a child and being content with the love of her husband. One day as I was reading, I got caught up in Hannah's prayer. She said, "If you give me a son, then I will give him to you all the days of his life." At that moment I realized that God didn't need Hannah to dedicate Samuel to His service. God wanted Hannah to be willing to give up the child. Hannah was desperate—so desperate that she was willing to give that child right back to God.

I too was desperate, scared, and in anguish. I felt convicted. I had spent seven months filling out paperwork, hoping that this whole thing would work out, but I had never committed the process to God. Instead, I was acting like a victim of my infertility and focused on what could have been rather than the beautiful gift God was giving me now. By His grace, I slowly stopped comparing my situation to everyone else's and started seeing what an amazing gift God was giving us through adoption. After all, we are God's adopted children, and I was blessed to get a miniscule glimpse into that type of love.

Once the home study paperwork was submitted, we had to go through a few interviews with our case manager. She explained our options.

"The wait time for couples in Illinois averages three to five years," she told us as we sat on a loveseat in her office. Immediately I felt the tears well up behind my eyes. *Three to five years? We're already one full year in. I can't wait another three to five years.*

"Although, I have had some couples use an advocate. Their wait time tends to be one to two years," she added.

"Yes, let's go with that option!" I said quickly. My husband, always the practical one, asked what all that entailed.

"Well, it means you might adopt a child from another state, which will mean traveling to that state and staying there until your adoption is approved and you can bring the baby home. The cost is also considerably different."

We went home and discussed all of our options. We also contacted a national Christian adoption agency and talked to them on the phone. Ultimately, we decided to use an advocate. We put together a profile book, which would give expectant mothers a glance into our lives. It included our background information, lots of photos, and answers to basic parenting questions so that the moms would have an idea of whom they were choosing for their baby. Once the profile was complete, we were in the "sit-and-wait" phase of adoption. Some families stay at this stage for a few weeks and others for years. There is no way to know how long it will be before you are chosen as an adoptive family.

During this time, we received emails from our advocate about potential adoptive cases. When we received an email, we prayed, talked, and decided if we wanted the adoption agency to show our book to the mother. Each week we heard a new story, talked for a few days and decided "yes, let's pursue this" or "no, this one doesn't seem right." We emailed our advocate and shared our decision, she passed our book along to the pregnant mother, and then we waited to hear if the mom chose us. It felt like we were living email to email, dreaming of possibilities, getting attached to various situations, and finding out that once again we were not the chosen family. At the beginning, we were optimistic and patient. Rejection was expected but never easy. There were a couple of cases that were harder than others. There were many tear-filled nights, but I kept holding on to the fact that God is good and He had a plan.

At the beginning of August, four months into this phase of the journey, I returned to teaching high school Family and Consumer Sciences. I reminded my principal that we were adopting, so there was a chance I would need to take a leave of absence at some point in the school year. Unlike a biological pregnancy, there was no clear timeline. Some of the adoption cases had mothers that were due in one week and others were only three months into their pregnancy.

On the third day of school, my phone rang in the middle of fourth period. I normally have my phone on silent, but apparently had forgotten to mute it that day. I went to silence the call and saw that it was our adoption caseworker. My high school students were finishing a pre-test, and I had an aide in the classroom, so I stepped into the closet of my classroom to take the call. She told me that an expectant mom looked at our profile and chose us to be the adoptive parents of her baby.

"Excuse me?" I said. *This couldn't be real*, I thought. I assumed she was calling to verify a fact in our bio or to ask if we had made a decision on the email we had received the night before.

"You've been chosen!" she said excitedly. "The expectant mom would like to speak with you before making it official, but she said your profile stood out from the others. She thinks you are the right family for her baby."

The next night we talked on the phone with Noel.* She told us that she was expecting a baby girl in mid-September, just five weeks away. We talked for about half an hour and everything clicked into place. She asked if we would use the name Hope, and we thought that sounded perfect after the journey we had been through. She was easy to talk to and incredibly kind. We learned a little about her family and her hopes for her baby.

On Thursday we signed papers and faxed them to her lawyer. We learned that we would owe a large sum of money in a few days since the birth was coming up so quickly. Typically, a deposit is due when papers are signed and the rest of the payment is due one month before birth. Since her baby was due in 5 weeks, the entire sum would be due in a matter of days.

Our adoption training had prepared us for this possibility and God had already provided a large portion of the money. Eight years earlier, before I had even met David, I bought an old house. When we moved to Illinois, we sold the house, and the equity provided most of what we needed; however, we were still seven thousand dollars short. All week long we looked into loans and grants. David and I called our parents and grandparents, and they were more than willing to help, but the logistics of getting the money from one account to another in time was a problem. We prayed about it, but we had no clue how we were going to wire the full amount by the deadline.

The morning the money was due, I woke up to get ready for school. I decided to check our bank account to be sure of the exact amount we needed. When I opened the app on my phone, my jaw dropped. Overnight $7,117 had been deposited into our account. It was the excess money from my student loan for my doctoral program. Normally I signed the paperwork to return the excess but in the chaos of starting the school year, I had forgotten to fill out the form. That oversight happened a month earlier, before we even knew about this baby. God knew what we would need and He gave us the money at the exact right moment.

We spent the weekend getting prepared for the baby by buying a few outfits, a crib, and other necessities. That Monday there was a historical solar eclipse and our town was in the area with the longest total eclipse, which meant a lot of traffic and tourists. My school chose to close for the day, so I was home with David. We went outside and witnessed the eclipse with our neighbors. As the sun was reappearing, Noel called me. She was at the doctor because she was experiencing complications, and she had some bad news. My heart dropped.

"Please don't be mad at me, but my doctor says it's a boy," she said in a rush.

It took me a second to realize what she meant. I assured her that we were happy with whatever God gave us. She sighed with relief and said that she was afraid we would change our minds. I told her there was no chance of that happening!

She told us that her doctors were monitoring her closely because she was losing fluid. She said there was a chance she would have an emergency c-section that evening.

"I'm sorry, what was that?" I asked.

"I think I'm going to deliver the baby tonight," she answered.

As the eclipse ended, we went into the house to pack our bags. Our caseworker assured us that this happened all the time and it would definitely be a few more weeks. Noel called me later that night to say that she was doing better and her doctor was able to get her stabilized. She had a follow-up appointment Thursday morning. At that appointment they would schedule her c-section.

We were anxious about the health of Noel and her baby, but ultimately, God gave us both a lot of peace. We went about our normal routine, but the packed suitcases stayed at the foot of the bed. Thursday morning, Noel called me in the middle of my first period. I was expecting her call and I had told my students I would need to take it. She let me know that her fluids were dropping rapidly and they were rushing her into delivery! This meant it was time to grab the suitcase and travel the 16 hours to the hospital.

God set everything in motion. Our bags were already packed and David was able to pick me up at school on the way. The day before, my long-term sub had shadowed me all day, so she knew what to expect. I had just signed paperwork for my maternity leave, so I didn't have to worry about getting everything sorted out while I was away. One week earlier we learned we had been chosen as parents and today it was happening! About three hours later while we were driving through Tennessee, we got the call that the baby had been born.

They asked us what they should name him, and we told them Andrew. Somehow the name got lost in the process and the official name on his birth certificate was "Baby Boy."

We got to the hospital around eleven that night and as we walked in, all I could think was *don't faint*. Since it was after visiting hours, a security guard had to escort us to the maternity ward. He tried making small talk with us on the elevator, but he quickly realized that we couldn't reciprocate.

We were given security badges and greeted by Noel's family. Her great-aunts were in the room with her, and they were sitting in the corner holding the most precious baby. I was overwhelmed and awkward. I was walking in to meet strangers who were simultaneously a few of the most important people in my life. Noel's aunt stood up and carried Baby Boy over to me. I took him into my arms and admired his handsome squished up face and head full of hair.

I wish I had words to describe meeting him for the first time, but all I really remember is that our smiles were huge and our hearts were full. I was holding a miracle. When I underwent infertility treatments, the doctor had said, "The odds of you becoming a mom are nearly impossible." She clearly meant the odds of me having a biological child were low, but it still affected me in a negative way. Thankfully I serve a God who does the impossible. I was no longer a victim of infertility. I was the recipient of a good and perfect gift directly from God.

Our little man needed to spend some time in the NICU and as Noel recovered from delivery, we were able to spend precious time getting to know our baby's birth mom. The day she was discharged she signed papers that gave us the biggest gift a person can give—her baby boy. We sat in the hallway waiting for her lawyer to meet with us, and I kept thinking about John 3:16 "For God so loved the world that He gave His only begotten Son." I can't imagine what it is like to give a child to another family, but I am so grateful for her gift.

We were hoping it would be a five-day NICU stay for Andrew, but we learned it would be three weeks. We made hotel arrangements and settled into our new normal. We spent every moment at the hospital and had many sleepless nights. We lived in hospital mode while the rest of the world went on without us. We caught glimpses of news here and there between rushing out for food and giving our parents updates. At the ten-day mark, a hurricane was threatening the state. The store shelves were empty and gas supplies were dwindling. We prepared to hunker down by buying water and keeping our gas tank full. We had both grown up in the Midwest, so we had no clue how to prepare for a hurricane.

By God's grace, Andrew improved faster than anticipated and would be discharged after only 13 days in the NICU, three days before the hurricane was expected to hit. My mom flew in the day before he was discharged, so she was there to help us on his first night out of the hospital. Since we would have to transport Andrew to another state to go home, we were waiting for word from the courts to approve our interstate travel. This process typically takes six to ten days, but one day later we got word that we could leave the state due to the impending natural disaster.

We were torn between staying and possibly experiencing a hurricane or driving home. If we headed home, we would be leaving Mom behind since her flight to Missouri wasn't scheduled for another few days and there was no room in our small car for her. Ultimately, we decided to drive back to Illinois to avoid the storm, leaving Mom to fend for herself in Florida. God took care of getting Mom home by giving her the last seat available on a flight that night. We drove out of Florida in bumper-to-bumper traffic with throngs of people trying to get out before the storm.

The next day we made it back to Illinois and we slowly adjusted to being a family of three. God had given us a miracle. When I look back at the process as a whole, I can see God's goodness in every intricate detail. Through this whole process I kept going back to the song "Teach Me, Lord, to Wait" by Stuart Hamblen based on Isaiah 40:31. My favorite lyrics are as follows:

Teach me, Lord, to wait—down on my knees.
Till in your own good time you'll answer my pleas.
Teach me not to rely on what others do.
But to wait in prayer for an answer from you.
(Hamblen, 1953)

We named Andrew after the disciple in the Bible because the few times that Andrew is mentioned in the gospels, he is bringing people to Jesus. That is exactly what my son did for me. I thought I knew what it meant to follow God and to give my entire life to Him, but the adoption journey took me to the foot of the cross.

The journey of adopting Andrew sent me down to my knees, waiting on God's timing. I cried out to God begging for a child much like Hannah had done in the temple. He loves me enough to weave together a story that not only ended with the best gift of being a mom, but it also gently pushed me to grow in my faith. I didn't need Google to get me through the process. I only needed the everlasting arms of God.

REFERENCES

Hamblen, S. (1953). Teach Me, Lord, to Wait. [Song]. Hamblen Music Co.

*Name changed

CHAPTER THREE

DO YOU HAVE PLANS?

By Kelsey Grant

"Twins," I murmured to myself, smiling. I took the small cotton socks hanging on the Walmart rack and gently rubbed them between my fingers, completely unaware of anyone else around me. I grabbed two pairs with camouflage print and hurried to the register.

My husband, Dan, had not been able to attend my first pregnancy appointment or the second one either. He was working deep in the pit of the steel plant, so I found my own way to the doctor's office and promised to tell him all the details when he arrived home. As the ultrasound technician pushed her slimy tool all over my belly, I held my breath. The first appointment revealed I was carrying a tiny bean-sized human being in my womb. What would she see this time? A beating heart and four limbs, I hoped.

"You know there's two in there, right?" The technician smiled as if I had already known somehow. Time froze. *Was this a joke? Could she not see the image very well? Whose idea was this anyway?* I plastered on the smile I wear when I'm uncomfortable and not sure how to respond. "Wow, twins . . . " My voice trailed off.

I left the appointment carrying a small black and white printout of two primordial blobs floating in black space. My sweaty grip was making the paper soft. My brain felt like the black space in the ultra-sound. *I had wanted one baby but how on earth would I care for two? What would Dan say?*

"They're cute, but why did you buy two pairs of the same socks?" He looked up at me, his face still smudged black and hair disheveled from work.

"Because . . . there's . . . TWO of them! We're having twins!" I smiled extra wide, hoping to coax a grin from him. I could see his brain was trying to process what his ears had just heard.

"Wow, twins . . . Okay, oh boy . . . " He smiled weakly and kissed me on the forehead. I could tell the idea was going to take some getting used to.

Two girls! It was hard to see, but the technician was sure. Dan and I settled on two beautiful girls' names: Claire and Libby. We bought lots of pink and proudly informed anyone who appeared halfway interested that I was carrying not one, but two baby girls.

A few weeks later at the next appointment, the technician appeared slightly confused. She gazed at her screen intently and I honed in on her furrowed brow, waiting for the grim news that I thought was sure to come.

"It's actually a boy and a girl. See there? That little thing, well, that means Baby A is actually a boy."

Claire was actually a Clarence!? *How could this be!* I had prayed for this, and I had even asked God if He could give me a little boy like Ralphie in *The Christmas Story*. I had found out I was pregnant right before Christmas and, for some unknown reason, my pregnant brain fixated on Ralphie and his black-rimmed glasses and toboggan. I wanted a little boy just like that. When I found out it was two girls, I told myself two healthy babies is more important than the gender. But now I began to envision what our growing family would really look like.

Proverbs 21:19 says, "Many are the plans in a man's heart, but it is the Lord's will that prevails." I had a lot of plans for my family:

visions of matching Easter outfits, little backpacks and lunch sacks on the first day of school and sending them off with a gentle push on a bicycle without training wheels. These daydreams kept me company during my lonely pregnancy. States away from my family and friends, I celebrated my good news with them online. I joined a local Moms of Multiples group and tried desperately to soak up every word of wisdom they shared from the battlefield. I borrowed heaps of parenting books from the library, studying intently for my ultimate test: Motherhood.

I faithfully attended each appointment, the promise of a new ultrasound picture being the ultimate incentive. The weeks melted together as sleeping, eating, and going to weekly appointments became my routine. No longer feeling like an independent woman with my own plans and desires, I was like a large living nest shielding and growing two new lives inside.

Weeks turned into months and then my high blood pressure made it impossible to carry the twins any longer. We scheduled the C-section at 35 weeks and I called my parents to let them know it was finally time. It could have been the drugs, or maybe it was the paralyzing nervousness, but the day of their birth is little more than a fuzzy memory. It was a blur of needle sticks, masked faces, a tugging feeling and then baby number one. "Hello, Benjamin Russell." Then another baby. "Hi, Libby Jean." I searched inside myself for the maternal instinct that would tell me to love and bond with these little strangers. It was there and it flooded through me like a warm light. The nurses let me hold them for a photo, and then whisked them away to be washed, tested, and measured. Although little, they appeared healthy, and we were admitted to our separate rooms to rest.

My breast milk came in quickly and soon I was pumping full bottles every couple of hours. The nurses told me the more I could be near them, the better my milk would come in. How I loved to gaze at their fragile wrinkled forms in their separate acrylic boxes. Ben had Strep B, but it would be easily treated with antibiotics. Libby's lungs were a little underdeveloped, but she should be just fine. I was exhausted but satisfied that the hardest part was over.

On the third day the NICU nurse called my hospital room. "Come quickly, please. Libby's heart rate is going down and we have paged the doctor." Dan rushed me downstairs in my wheelchair. They had already closed the curtain to Libby's room so we had to wait in Ben's room. I saw the shadows of frantic doctors and nurses moving behind the blue drapes. Someone shoved the recliner from the room into the hallway. *I had just been rocking her in that chair this morning*, I thought to myself. I sat next to Ben in his box while Dan and I stared at the commotion across the hall. *Was I watching our new family of four become a family of three?* Plastic wrappers that protected syringes and gauze were strewn carelessly on the floor as the NICU team desperately tried to revive Libby. She was in cardiac arrest and the pediatric cardiologist was not at this hospital; he was at the university hospital a few miles away.

I should pause and tell you that at this point in my life my faith in God was like a puny, untrained muscle. Sure, I had accepted Jesus into my heart at age seven, and my mom had faithfully brought me to church every Sunday. But I was living life on my own terms these days. Jesus was someone I would think about when I got older, and a little closer to death. Suddenly death appeared imminent, ready to take my baby girl, and I was not ready. I did not have any words to pray, no requests for miracles came out of my dry mouth.

Libby's NICU pediatrician was a man with a bulging prayer muscle. He knew just what to pray and called his family and church far away in Belize to request their urgent prayers as well. Here was a man I had just met, yet he sprang into action both physically and spiritually to save my daughter. I informed my own parents of the abrupt turn of events and asked them to meet me with a change of clothes. I did not recognize my own voice in the hollow flat tone I heard on the phone. My mom called her own church to ask for prayer and soon we had people in several states and two different countries lifting up prayers for our daughter.

Libby was loaded in an ambulance and rushed to the university hospital in downtown Birmingham. In the midst of this chaos, I needed to be discharged from the hospital while leaving my other newborn quietly waiting for me in his room. The ripping pain of the C-Section incision brought tears to my eyes and I wondered if I would survive waddling downtown to the other hospital to find my daughter. *Would she even be alive when I got there, or would it be too late?*

On the way downtown, Dan's cell phone rang. We both froze and looked at each other, not sure whether we wanted to know the information coming from the other end. He picked it up.

"Mr. Grant, this is the NICU doctor from UAB. Libby is a very sick baby. We would like to try an experimental treatment on her that could save her brain function while we try to find and stabilize the pulse and examine the damage from the code event. We want to put her on a cooling bed and bring her temperature down for a few days. We need to have your permission right now."

Stunned, we opened our mouths, but no words came out. Dan finally managed to ask, "Would you use this treatment on your own child?" When the doctor emphatically answered yes, we agreed and hoped for the best. I wish I could write that we prayed for the best, but my first thoughts were not on the sovereign God in control of all things, but on my own limitations and inability to control the situation.

As the days turned to weeks in the hospital, each new piece of information about Libby's condition was grim. She was swelling up like a balloon and an exploratory surgery revealed one-third of her stomach tissue had died and needed to be removed. She would need a feeding tube and maybe a colostomy bag. She had a brain hemorrhage and swelling and might need a shunt to drain the fluid. The fluid in her body was not responding to the diuretics and she required dialysis. She was also intubated and not even close to breathing on her own.

All the daydreams I had savored over the past months began slipping through my fingers. *Would I need to find special clothing for her to wear over her medical devices? They do not make matching Easter outfits like that. Would she ever ride a bicycle or would her mode of transportation forever be a wheelchair?* Instead of running into the arms of the One who could comfort me with His perfect peace, I ran the other way. I ran into the dark tunnel called "Why Me?". Inside that black gaping hole were thoughts like *I'm not even a drug addict and my baby has all these problems. What did I ever do to you, God?*

Bitterness bubbled up in the back of my throat like bile. I shrank away from the many compassionate shoulder-pats and consoling looks. I retreated into my own dark, brooding thoughts while failing to acknowledge I had a husband and a son who needed me to care about them. I had family and friends that were concerned about me. The praying doctor came by with his wife and even brought a meal from Olive Garden to our hospital room one evening. Yet, all of this still failed to soften my heart towards the Lord who had carefully placed this loving safety net of praying believers around me.

All I wanted to do was hide and be alone with my own thoughts, not have to give updates to friends and family, or try to smile and nod optimistically at the doctors and nurses. The only privacy I found was in the nursing room of the hospital. Also used as a storage closet, the boxes of supplies and trash overflowed around me. I huddled in the hard plastic chair, trying to attach the breast pump through blurry tears. The last stale sips of coffee in Styrofoam cups stayed in the trashcan for the weeks we were there, never emptied. I can still conjure this smell in my memory today and perhaps it reminds me of my own reeking bitterness. I was in self-preservation mode and as my world spun chaotically around me, I searched desperately for a way to make life manageable. I would like to say that this is the point in my story that I finally took refuge under the Wing of the Almighty, but instead I found solace in any substance or prescription I could find.

After 63 days in the hospital, Libby was finally able to come home. I relished holding her in my arms with no IVs or sensors attached and dressing her in real clothes. If one could look past her jaundiced skin and Frankenstein stitches and my bloodshot, bag-ridden eyes, we almost looked like a regular mom and baby. Fresh with new hope, I attempted to master the regimen that would be part of our daily lives. It was terrifying at first to watch her wretch up the formula and medicine cocktail that I too-aggressively poured into her feeding tube. Over time, I learned to draw miniscule droppers of medicine, to work around her incision sites at every diaper change or bath, and to operate the button on her belly where she received her nourishment. I felt like I was watching someone else's life. The days were lonely and stressful as I tried to manage two infants at every doctor appointment and errand.

Believing we needed to be closer to family, we moved to Houston armed with a stack of referrals for all the best pediatric specialists at Texas Children's Hospital. We were ready to turn a new leaf and start over. You might think that a move and change of pace were what I needed to reconnect with the Lord and reignite the flame of my faith. Unfortunately, the isolation of living in a huge metropolis threw me into a deeper depression and I continued my headstrong journey into the pit of victimhood and resentment. To combat these unbearable feelings, I cloaked myself in the kind of apathy only too much Xanax can provide. I realize now that my anger was really fear and sadness. Mourning a broken dream was more than I could stand, and I lashed out at those closest to me, retreating behind a thick cloak of anti-anxiety medication.

In the meantime, my relationship with my husband was crumbling. Instead of supporting and caring for Dan, I abandoned him, believing he was capable of handling his own pain. Lost in my own self-absorption, I neglected to care for my husband in the way that I should have. He shouldered the responsibility of supporting our family financially while also trying to sort out insurance bills, medications, and other family matters. It was a load too big to bear alone. Unattended for too long, our marriage was at the point where divorce seemed like the only viable option. My own selfishness left me unable to realize that I was the reason behind the demise of our marriage. "You've checked out as a mom and a wife. Are you ever coming back? You hardly ever interact with us or even leave the house," he said. Dan's words stung. *Me, checked out?* All this time I had been buying into my own lie that I was the one holding things together. Reality hit me like a wrecking ball. "We need some help." With that simple admission to myself and Dan, a crack began to form on the wall around my heart. I watched in amazement as Dan put aside his own ego to forgive me and care for me with fresh tenderness. He had all the right in the world to hold my indiscretions over my head, but he took the high road of humility and gentleness. We resolved to begin attending church again, and slowly the Lord began to chip away at my hardened heart.

I started to have a change in perspective. It was gradual, but noticeable. I accepted the truth that even if nothing else went right for the rest of my life, I had my Savior Jesus Christ and I would spend eternity with Him. Gratitude began seeping out of my pores. There had never been a day in my life that I had to go without, for the Lord tended to my every need. We lived in an area with outstanding medical care and I did not have to juggle time off work to take the twins to their appointments. I had a husband and family who loved me, and a miraculous baby girl who had defied all the odds. It is hard to wallow in self-pity once you begin to count your blessings.

Even with a shunt and thick glasses, Libby has been able to thrive in school alongside her brother and friends. Her beautiful faith in Jesus and the way it impacts those around her shows me that God indeed has a special purpose for all our suffering. Although warned by the doctors about the possibility of leg braces, Libby has never even had a limp. Her feeding tube was removed weeks after it was put in which was an astonishing victory.

We have had many scares with Libby over the years. The shunt she wears on the back of her head for hydrocephalus has malfunctioned many times. Each time we go to the hospital I am amazed at all the ways God provides for us. From finding a parking spot in a full garage, to being able to bypass seemingly unavoidable surgeries, the Lord has lavished His goodness on our family at every turn.

In March of last year, we had another medical scare which was not the normal shunt malfunction. This time, Libby was suddenly, mysteriously, and completely losing her eyesight. The doctors were dismissive at first of her condition and suggested that maybe she just needed new glasses. As her condition worsened, their indifference changed to bewilderment, and we were given the arduous task of waiting patiently for test results. I remember asking Dan, "Will we need to move closer to a school for the blind?" I was imagining a future of Seeing Eye dogs, canes, and learning Braille. I could feel myself turning back to fear and anger. But those old ways no longer served me well and God was not finished with me yet. This time with the help of the Holy Spirit, I was able to summon the faith and strength to praise Him in the midst of my suffering. I was able to see my blessings in real time and be a light to those around me. His relentless grace and mercy pursued and found me once again. Although her sight eventually returned, the looming uncertainty of another episode sometimes makes my spiritual knees quake. But 2 Timothy 1:7 reminds me, "For God has not given us a spirit of fear, but of power, love, and self-control." His power gives me the strength to love Him and others, and the self-control to avoid spiraling destructive thoughts.

I believe both the truth that all good things come from God, and also that He gives and He takes away. I had to learn that Libby was never mine to "own" in the first place, but a gift from God to treasure, protect, and care for while we have her. Sometimes mothers get that gift for many years but sometimes they do not. When I returned to reading the Word and recounted the goodness of God and all of the promises He has kept, I received strength and encouragement. Even though I had to surrender control of my most precious possession to Him, I have felt the supernaturally perfect peace that comes when we remain steadfast in our faith. What that practically looks like is not asking "Why me?" anymore. It means looking for things to be thankful for when I don't see them right away. It means not taking out my frustration on the people around me. It means not trying to hide from the pain through distractions. Sometimes it just means physically putting my hands out to Him in prayer saying, "Here you go, God. I don't understand this and I need you." God can handle it when we pour out our despair and anguish to Him. He does not chastise us but understands our feelings. Through His life on earth, Jesus understands suffering like none other. Sometimes I have to surrender over and over again, but when I do, God shows me that He knows me intimately, cares for me deeply, and will meet me in my brokenness.

It is difficult to truly convey the change God has made in me. In the old days I would turn up my beloved heavy metal to maximum volume, beat thumping in my chest, trying to drown out anything but my blinding rage. Now, I find myself drawn to praise hymns and worship ballads. I realize that even if I used every breath I have for the rest of my life praising the Lord, it would not give Him all the glory He deserves. Instead of searching for solace in the empty void of social media or Netflix, I can open up God's Word and find encouragement and life-giving truth. The old me would probably laugh at the new me today, and maybe even whisper "Ned Flanders" under my breath, but the new me finds less value in the opinion of others.

There is a living God who is constantly working through the struggles of our lives so that they can be used for our good and His glory. Whatever season of suffering you are in, do not let it go to waste. Give your circumstances to a God who can lovingly weave together all things for the good of those who love Him. Resist the world's mantra that you are a victim and entitled to search for your happiness at any cost. True comfort can only come from Him whose burden is light and whose yoke is easy.

I realize these words are much easier to type than to put into practice. Learning to love God, my husband and children, and myself means seeing love as an action and not a feeling. Love means sometimes having to sacrifice my time and comfort even when I am tired and overwhelmed in order to care for others. Love means praising God even when everything around me seems out of control. Love means sharing my story with you even when it is painful. I invite you to lay your burdens down at the door and spend some time with the One who knows you intimately and loves you madly. I promise He has just what you need.

CHAPTER FOUR

UNDONE

By Terah K. Hensley

Completely undone. That's where I'm at today, sitting down in my home office, preparing to share this story with parents who are waiting for their children to arrive. As I prayed for guidance on what to share and how to tell this part of our family's story, I felt an intense tenderness toward the readers who have grabbed this book looking for hope. For those of you who are in the middle of the waiting game. You're in the wilderness of faith, wandering around and waiting to come into the Promised Land. You trust God, He's brought you this far, but you're wondering *where did He go? How long will you wait? What is the purpose of all this wandering?* You're tired and your heart hurts and sometimes the sight of children stings so sharply all you can do is close your eyes and breathe through the pain. If this sounds familiar, I see you. I know the pain of birth announcements, pregnancy complaints, and confusion about my own body. You're not alone. There are so many of us who must walk this journey and I can't pretend to know all the reasons why. I do know one thing though–that you are blessed. You are blessed right now, in the waiting. God is writing a story with your life and I promise you, it is more beautiful than the one you could write for yourself.

I met my husband, Heath, when we were both thirteen years old. We didn't know anything about real love, but we gave our hearts to each other at that young age and we never got them back. We went from being middle school sweethearts to prom king and queen our senior year of high school. In many ways it was like living in a fairy tale. We talked about getting married after college and did a lot of dreaming about our future together.

Shortly after graduating from high school, my younger brother was killed in a car crash. My brother and I were extremely close and it was the first time I had ever experienced pain so intense that I forgot how to breathe. We left for college a month later and Heath became my rock. I share this side story because I want you to know that the pain of loss, which came into my life like a thief in the night . . . the pain that left me deaf and crumpled on the floor drowning in my own snot and tears, followed by *years* of God putting my heart back together . . . it couldn't hold a candle to the pain of infertility. Please hear that and let it validate your brokenness.

Infertility doesn't come into our lives as fast and furious as something like a sudden loss or a diagnosis with a bad prognosis, and so I don't think it gets the respect it deserves. It is a monster. It haunts us in the quiet places and steals our joy, slowly and painfully carving up our hearts into a mess we don't recognize. Jealousy and bitterness take hold and we must fight to keep ourselves afloat, to smile. The truth is, we are in mourning. We have experienced major loss. We *have* received a diagnosis and the prognosis does not look good. Infertility is so misunderstood by the world around us. And yet, you are blessed to share in this suffering. You understand this pain and you will have a richer story to tell because of it. Keep fighting to smile, fight to believe and to trust that God is fighting for you while you wander through the wilderness. Stand firm and remember who He is. He will deliver you from this foe.

When God delivered the Israelites from slavery in Egypt and led them to the Red Sea, the people cried out in fear at the pursuing

Egyptian army. Moses answered the people, "Do not be afraid. Stand firm and you will see the deliverance the Lord will bring you today. The Egyptians you see today you will never see again. The Lord will fight for you; You need only to be still" (Exodus. 14:13-14).

In my early twenties, I would find myself dreaming of the next chapter in my life. I loved to engage Heath in these dreams and we would spend hours discussing our hopes for our future together. We often talked about our kids. *What would we teach them? Where would we take them on family vacations?* And of course, *how old did they need to be to start reading Harry Potter?* Since we didn't actually have any kids yet, we thought we wanted half a football teams' worth. We loved kids! We had nieces and nephews to love on, and being around children was so life giving for me that I became an elementary school teacher so I could spend my days with children. When we finally got married (at the age of 21) we saw each other as our unborn children's mother and father. There was no question at that point about whether or not there would be children in our family at all.

What happened next felt like a complete derailment of our lives. Heath and I had been making our own plans for many years and things were going exactly the way we wanted them to. If a problem arose, we fixed it together and kept moving forward. We had so much perceived control over our lives and it felt good. We were making all of our dreams come true and I'm sad to say that we didn't feel the need to rely on God very much. There was nothing happening in our lives that if He didn't show up, we would've noticed. This is one of the many reasons why our years of infertility were a true blessing. Not the "hashtag blessed" kind of blessing, but the hard kind–the real kind. The kind of blessing that knocks you flat on your face because you have been relying on your own strength to get through life instead of His and you desperately need a wakeup call. It's something to remind you that you are not, in fact, in control at all and the only way to receive the Father's good gifts is to ask Him. Ask Him to show up for you, because you know that if He doesn't, there is no hope left. When you find yourself on your knees, tears stained down your cheeks, with little-to-no strength left praying, "Father, if you do not make this happen, this dream is dead," then you are in a good place. A hard place, absolutely, but a good place. Twentieth-century Dutch priest Henri Nouwen prayed it like this,

> Dear God,
> I so much want to be in control.
> I want to be the master of my own destiny.
> Still I know that you are saying:
> "Let me take you by the hand and lead you.
> Accept my love
> And trust that where I will bring you,
> The deepest desires of your heart will be fulfilled."
> Lord, open my hands to receive your gift of love.
> Amen.[1]

While Heath and I were trying to grow our family, I found myself surrounded by co-workers who planned their pregnancies, with great accuracy, to deliver their babies in May, so they could enjoy the summer off with the new baby. Many of our closest friends started building their families with so much ease that some even made sure not to conceive during certain months so they didn't have a holiday birthday in their family! One baby shower turned into two and then four and then when our friends started to announce the pregnancies of their second babies, it started to cut my heart deeply. To add insult to injury, Heath's sister, who is *ten* years older than us, found out by surprise that she was expecting her sixth child. We were happy for our friends and family and they are all wonderful people, but I can hardly put into words how difficult this season was for us. If there is a more tender topic for couples than unmet parental longings, I don't know what it is.

We were fortunate to have formed a deep friendship with another couple experiencing the same struggle and, for several years, we were a great comfort to one another as we celebrated the births of our friends' children together with our empty wombs and crib-less homes. The richness and the gift of that friendship has transcended many seasons since that time and there will always be a strong connection that needs no explanation between the four of us. This was an amazing blessing God gave us during the waiting that wouldn't have happened had we been allowed to make our own plans. The birth of this friendship was the fulfillment of a desire we had as a young couple for new friends. We had prayed often for God to connect us with another couple that would become family. We were looking for soulmate friends to raise our families together, be there for each other no matter what, and grow old with. We desperately wanted that kind of friendship in our lives and it was fulfilled through our shared suffering with infertility. God doesn't always cause our struggles, but He does promise to use them for our good. "And we know that *in all things* God works for the good of those who love him, who have been called according to his purpose." Romans 8:28 (emphasis added).

God really is good. He is for us and He is working out a plan for our lives that will blow our minds. When we believe that He knows us better than we know ourselves, that He sees the real "us" beneath the self-centeredness and knows how to call that version of us to full life, we will surrender. Our fears of what He may call us to will be held in perfect tension with our trust and we will have courage. We will release the tight grip we have on our future and with open hands we will boldly proclaim, "Your will, not mine." Ask the creator of the universe to build your family the way He sees fit and then trust that He knows what He's doing. It took about a year and a half for me to pray that way, but once I did, it was liberating. I could honestly pray that "Whatever family you want for me, that's the one I want." I definitely prayed it afraid of the ways He might answer it, but I trusted that He knew best.

It was about that time that we decided to stop seeing doctors about my reproductive situation. We hadn't made it very far down the infertility medical road, but I had been diagnosed with PCOS (poly-cystic ovarian syndrome) and was about to hit the two-year mark without having a menstrual cycle. We were told initially that this condition was very common and would be an easy fix with some simple medication. It didn't work. After lots of confusion, several doctors and various medications, we still couldn't make my stubborn ovaries release those precious eggs. It felt like this was happening intentionally. I started to dig through my Bible and read every verse that spoke about wombs. It seemed pretty clear to me that God was very involved in the opening and the closing of wombs to fulfill His purposes and so I believed mine was closed for a reason. I thought maybe one day God would open it for me, but for the time being, this was an answer that allowed me to move on with hope.

Heath and I always wanted our family to be a blend of our own biological children and children through adoption. We thought our stadium-sized family would be as colorful as Joseph's coat, and as eclectic as heaven. We envisioned many cultures, abilities, and all the different shades of God's image-bearers under one (giant) roof! Of course, we were young and dumb and that would take an entire theme park staff to help us corral and feed the animals we would call our children. But what mattered was that our hearts were open and we always wanted to adopt. It was, in our minds, going to be second. We would have all the babies we wanted and then we would start adopting the rest! God so graciously had mercy on us. He knew that adoption would be part of our story and that it was never going to be second. Society seems to place it second, but God puts it first. It is not second best to having children of your own body, it is not plan B, and it is not the last resort. It is and always was God's plan A for us. Adoption is how He redeemed you and me and we are daughters and sons of a King who will make all things new. Joseph adopted Jesus and raised Him as his own. God adopted us because He loves us and wants us to be His children and then tells us to call him, "Abba, Papa." Adoption is first. And God was putting it where it belonged in our family: first.

For us, the mental flip we made to adopting our firstborn child was pretty easy. As we went through the adoption process, we had complete faith that God was guiding us to a baby already growing inside a mother's womb. The local agency we worked with told us that it usually takes up to six months to complete all of the necessary paperwork and appointments. This was disheartening to hear, knowing that there was a barrier of that length to even begin to wait. Once we were officially waiting to be matched with a birthmother, adoption would likely happen within two years. That's 30 months altogether and we had already waited that long hoping to become pregnant. We felt defeated before we even began, but we knew God was leading us down this path. We made a goal to finish all of the paperwork and meet every requirement in three months instead of six.

As we set out reading the required parenting books and writing book reports (yes, seriously), our friends continued to conceive with ease and have their babies without being asked to write a single book report. They didn't have to get a financial background check, schedule monthly home-visits from state-licensed social workers or give an in-depth presentation of their parenting goals. They didn't have to save a million dollars (these are rough numbers) or get a doctor to perform a physical exam and sign off that they are healthy enough to raise children. I was thrilled to be adopting, but I wondered why I had to jump through so many hoops to get my baby home while others didn't. I was becoming bitter about the whole process.

Even though I knew we were walking the path that God laid before us, I kept looking back. I would let my heart slip into despair and try to stuff down the cries of my soul for Heath and I to make a baby together. Remember how we met? Just thirteen, high-school sweethearts, the fairy-tale young love strengthened by loss and by Heath's steadfast love for me in the aftermath? My rock, the one who stood by my side as I ran from God and lifted me up in his prayers? The boy who has shown me nothing but the love of Christ since the day we met. That boy, now a man. My faithful husband . . . how could *we* not be able to have a baby? We have loved each other forever and it felt like a tragedy to me that strangers could conceive during a one-night stand, but we may never get to see a baby who's a combination of the two of us. It broke my heart and I let God know, from the deepest, most secret parts of me, that I still wanted that gift.

We started the adoption paperwork on January 1st and by March 31st, we submitted the final document to our agency. We nailed it, as we like to say, and we were ready to be matched! The only thing left to do was to save the rest of the money that we'd need once we were chosen. It was no small amount and we were told that if we didn't have it when the baby was born, the baby wouldn't be ours. Since most couples wait a year or two to be matched, they told us we'd have plenty of time to save. But I felt in my heart that we better get our hands on those funds right away. We had been saving every single penny for months and even held a yard sale where we sold pretty much every loose item in our home. Family and friends donated to the cause and we were getting closer to having the final amount. I can still remember that during this time my (amazing) mother-in-law asked us to bring French bread to a family gathering and the expense of it (probably a few dollars) brought me to tears. I felt an urgency to get the money ready and I was starting to lose hope that we would have what we needed in time.

This is the point in our story when God started speaking loud and clear. All along it was like we had been following signs and proceeding with what brought us peace. We felt our way along the dimly lit path, only seeing one step ahead at a time and trusting that God was leading us toward His will for our family. But after our adoption profile went "live" it was like all of the lights came on. We could see clearly what our Father was up to and how He was engineering our family together with a design we never could have dreamed up on our own.

The very same day that we became officially "waiting" parents with the agency, we received an email from our tax accountant. Never in our lives had we received a tax return and on March 31st, moments after we dropped off the last remaining papers to our adoption agency, we opened the email. It stopped us in our tracks. It was a tax return for the *exact* amount we had left to save! God was not just speaking to us, He was shouting! It was confirmation that we were on the right path and it felt like a sweet reward for listening to the voice of our Father. We praised God and wrote the last check!

The very next day, I bled for the first time in nearly two years. My menstrual cycle was back without any doctors or medication. We couldn't believe the timing of it, but we knew that God had done it! He had closed my womb for a time to lead us to the child He had destined to be ours. Now that our adoption profile was in the mix, He opened my womb. I knew He was telling me that one day in our future He would let me carry a child for our family and my hope for that dream was restored.

I would love to say that I never doubted God again in the formation of our family and everything was rainbows and butterflies while we waited for things to play out, but that wasn't the case. I was still dealing with jealousy, anger, and bitterness. I was still struggling as the wait dragged on. A month went by and we heard nothing from the agency, then two, then three, then four. It was harder than I thought it was going to be and I decided to keep a journal to capture my state of being during that time. I want to share some of the things I wrote while waiting to become a mother.

I have entered a weird phase of waiting where I almost don't believe it is going to happen. Like . . . ever. That we'll never get picked. I think I still have a lot of anger about the unfairness of it. About not getting to control the baby's prenatal care and having to deal with the consequences. Sometimes I feel like I can't do this. Not because I can't love a child born of someone else, but because there are too many unknowns and it is exhausting me. How long will we wait? Will the baby be born healthy or premature or addicted to drugs? Will we bond okay? Will Heath and I still love our lives as much as we do now? It's just so much to think about. It's overwhelming. I want to be excited about waiting, about becoming a parent, but today, I am not feeling excited. I am feeling tired, faithless, and inadequate to do this. I purposefully avoid thinking about it, or talking about it. I don't want to paint the "nursery" and even have a hard time calling it that. I don't want to think about names and baby showers, and I think I must've been crazy looking at baby products on amazon, adding them to my secret baby registry like an expectant mother, like some kind of fraud. I was so pumped and happy when we were doing the paperwork, and now the longer the wait gets, the more I doubt it all. The more depressed I feel. I know this is a phase and I know it will pass. When I get down to the roots, I know that God is in control of it all, and I trust Him. If He wants me to have a certain child, then I want that child, even if I can't see things His way yet. Waiting is a hard game.

In some ways, I felt forgotten by God during this time. He had been so undeniably involved months earlier and now I couldn't sense His presence. It was like I was right back where I started, wandering through the wilderness, wondering when and if my God was ever going to deliver me from the pain of being childless. King David captured the mood of my heart with his opening lines of the thirteenth psalm; "How long, O Lord? Will you forget me forever?" Psalm 13:1a.

But I still had hope that the God of the Cosmos was going to come through for me and that He was going to form the most beautiful family out of our brokenness. It's His favorite thing to do! To save what is lost and make all things new. He redeems lives for Himself out of His steadfast love and His faithfulness. I had great hope that even if I didn't know where He went the past couple of months, that He was working out a plan for us. He was taking our brokenness and someone else's and was going to build something new out of the pieces–something God-breathed, divinely engineered, redeemed, restored, and saved by grace. He was going to do something that only He can do! By the end of Psalm 13 David's mourning had turned to exaltation; "But I have trusted in your steadfast love; my heart shall rejoice in your salvation. I will sing to the Lord because he has dealt bountifully with me" (Psalm 13:5-6).

I never had another menstrual cycle. The very first time my ovaries were back in business, God created a baby in me. It felt like the greatest gift! To have tried for so long to make this happen and then to be surprised by pregnancy was so sweet and undeserved. God had dealt bountifully with me!

We called the agency to tell them that we were expecting a baby on our own and to our shock, they told us that it would be best to remove our profile and wait until after our baby turned one year old to get back to adopting. I was having none of it. None. Of. It. I told them my story and explained to them that I was convinced there was a baby who belonged in our family, growing inside another's womb *right now*! I shared all that God had been teaching me about the construction of our family and I asked if we could still have our profile shown to birthmothers. They said that in over 25 years of operation they had never allowed a couple that became pregnant to continue with the adoption process. They said "natural age gaps" were best for families and we were welcome to come back in a couple of years. I implored them to make a way for us. They gathered the board of directors and discussed my request. A few days later they called to say that if God was telling me there is a baby for us right now, who are they to stand in the way of that match? The agency asked us to update our profile to let the birthmother know that we were expecting to deliver our own baby and told us that it may deter many birthmothers from choosing us. My reply? "That's okay! It won't deter ours." I don't know if I've ever been more confident about anything in my life.

A few weeks later, we got a phone call. It was a Thursday evening and Heath was on his way home from work pleading with God (as I later found out) to show him how to bring God glory. It was a phrase he had latched onto and the whole way home he repeated, "Show me, God, how to glorify you." When he walked through the front door, I was holding the phone on speaker and excitedly waved him over. Our adoption agent had just called as Heath was pulling into the driveway and said she had some news for us. "He's here! Tell us the news!" I squealed! Hope was rising in my chest and there was nothing I could do to stop it. "You've been matched with a birthmother!" she said. Heath and I held our breath for a few seconds and I don't remember what we said, but I know we were celebrating with praise and dancing! Our agent gave us a few moments and then grabbed our attention. "Also," she said, "the baby's due tomorrow!" I think our eyes grew three times their normal size and the tears just streamed down both of our faces. We found out later that one of the reasons our son's birthmother chose us was because we were expecting a child and she wanted her baby to have a sibling. What may have stopped others from choosing us actually drew her to us. God is so creative and so good.

Our baby, Solomon, was born a week later. Within that week, our friends and family dropped everything to come and help us prepare for the arrival of our son. They painted the nursery, built the crib and changing table, washed baby clothes, stocked formula and bottles in the kitchen, and made sure we had everything a baby needs. We went from having absolutely nothing to having more than enough in just a few days! It was incredible to see the outpouring of love and support from our community; it was yet another way God used all of the preceding hardships to bless us.

Almost six months later, we delivered our second child. Another son we named Elijah. After years of a baby drought in our house, it was now raining babies and we were so grateful. I don't think a day went by that first year that tears of joy didn't flow down my face. God had seen me, in all my pain and desire to be a mother, and He gave me not one, but *two* babies at the same time. Two little boys who would grow up to be the closest of brothers and do everything together. They would even be ready to read Harry Potter at the same time! God really knew how to make my heart sing and words couldn't express my joy, so most of the time I used my tears. Both of these babies were true miracles. How could God be so loving and so good to make sure that none of us missed each other in making our own plans? To Him be the glory for His perfect timing and His will for our family.

Years later, we were blessed with another surprise pregnancy but unfortunately that baby didn't survive the womb. God comforted us during that loss with the love and warmth of close friends and family who ministered to us in our sadness. A few months later, we were expecting again and this time I felt fearful of losing this baby too. We decided to keep the news close to home until we made it past the first trimester and at the twelve-week mark, we announced the good news to friends and family. We were all so happy for another baby to join our family! The very next day I started bleeding heavily and all of my worst fears began flooding my heart and mind. I begged God to heal me and save this baby that He had created. I texted all of our closest friends late at night and asked them to get up and pray for our baby's life. They did. The next morning the bleeding had stopped and we went to the doctor to check on the baby. The tech started the ultrasound and I held my breath. After a few moments she said, "There's the baby's heartbeat and I don't see any signs of bleeding." Heath immediately started crying, but I didn't trust the good news yet. "Is the baby going to be okay? Is the heart going to *keep* beating?" I asked. She assured me that everything looked exactly as it should at that stage. We met with the doctor and she had a lot of questions about the blood I saw the night before, almost as if she didn't believe I had been bleeding. There were zero signs of bleeding. Nothing was wrong and everything looked perfectly healthy. I knew that God had heard the cry of my heart and of His people and He had intervened. Six months later our beautiful daughter, Anna Kay, was born as healthy as could be and we brought our third miracle babe home.

At the time of this writing we have three little blessings who call us mom and dad. It isn't half a football team, we don't need a stadium to fit us all in, and we don't require any staff to help us corral and feed these animals, but we are so full. We are full of wonder and gratitude to the only One who has the power to create life. We are full of love for the little lives He has entrusted to us to raise. In His steadfast love and faithfulness, He brought us to a place of full surrender and then gave us everything we didn't even know we wanted in a family. Why? Because He cares for us. That is completely wild and it still brings me to a place of profound praise and thankfulness.

I don't know how long you will wait or who God will give you to love. I do believe that if you want to be a parent, you can be. If the Creator of the universe gave you a desire to love and to nurture children, you must trust Him with that desire. Open your heart and let God build your family the way He wants. Loosen your grip on the future and go to the One who has the power to create life. He sees you and He cares for you. As you continue to wait for His bountiful gifts, keep asking Him to do what He does best; to redeem what's broken and to save what's lost. "Be strong, and let your heart take courage, all you who wait for the Lord!" Psalm 31:24

REFERENCES

1. Nouwen, H. (2023, January 31). *A prayer*. Henri Nouwen Society. https://henrinouwen.org/meditations/a-prayer/

CHAPTER FIVE

SELAH: PAUSE, PONDER, AND PRAISE

By Lindsey Racz

I didn't necessarily dream of being a mom when I was little. As a girl, I spent a lot of time dreaming I would be a famous singer and practicing my skills with Mariah Carey's accompaniment. Or, I reasoned, I could also be a famous fashion designer out of Paris. Naturally, I practiced on my dolls by making dresses out of cut up socks and decorating them with marvelous puff paint and glitter designs.

FALLING APART

Somewhere between belting "Always Be My Baby" from my swing set and styling Barbie, my family fell apart.

My mom is a well-educated teacher from Michigan and my father was a folk musician with a propensity to drink. I don't blame my father for choosing alcohol over his family. Looking back, I can see that he had untreated pain through mental illness and trauma and the only way he knew to treat it was to numb it with drinking. He was a silly drunk, not a mean one. For that, I am thankful.

Sadly, due to his inability to hold a job, our family went under, financially and every other possible way. My hard-working mom just couldn't hold us together. I was nine when I realized that life is very scary. I must have subconsciously equated safety to family and the lack of family to danger. After my dad was out of the picture, I began to suffer sexual abuse at the hands of a family friend. I wasn't wrong in this early developmental association that families provide safety.

After my parents' divorce, my dad moved to a cabin in the woods and I missed him madly. At the same time, my only sister, who is eight years older, moved off to college. We quickly went from a household of four down to two. My mom and I remained. It seems that from that moment on, it was seared into my soul that I needed to re-establish a family of my own. I think this obsession escalated when my mom married an engineer. He and all three of his kids moved in with my mom and me. As an adult, I am so happy my stepdad came along—he has loved my mom well for the last 25 years. As a kid, however, it felt as if I had just lost my last remaining family member to this new guy. *Where did I belong?*

I can look back now and see my adolescent years as a desperate attempt to find someone who would show me I belonged. I was looking, even then, to create a family of my own. Although I never struggled academically and even graduated with honors, I did struggle to fit in. I didn't want the normal high school experience. I remember sitting in French class one day and overhearing girls discussing prom dresses; all I could think about was how I could get out of this God-forsaken place called high school, get married, and settle down into safety. I constantly fantasized about having a family of my own.

As a freshman and sophomore in high school, my hunger to belong and be loved led to promiscuity and heartache beyond words. At age 15, probably struggling with my own genetically linked and circumstantial clinical depression, I attempted to take my life. Shortly after that, God came after me hard. I like to think He looked down, saw my desperation, and pointed—"That one. That one isn't going to make it much longer on her own. I'm going in to get her." And He did.

THE RESCUE

It happened like this. A friend of mine, one of the wildest in our little friend group, suddenly announced to me one day, as we were primping in the school bathroom, that she wasn't going to cuss anymore. I remember looking at her and saying something classy like "why the **** not?" She explained that she had begun going to church. Something had changed about her through this experience, and she was now different, she said. I could see this difference.

She invited me to go to church with her. Relentlessly. I was a "no thank you" until that fateful day when I learned that Nathan went to her church. Nathan was cute and I thought that maybe he would be my husband someday. Husband plus babies equals a family of my own. I was in. I attended church for the first time on a Wednesday night in November. It was a service just for youth and it was packed! I was a sophomore and one month shy of turning 16. I was sexually active with my much older boyfriend and using marijuana and alcohol. But that night everything changed.

I don't remember what the sermon was about, but I do remember the feeling of my heart racing in my chest. The pastor spoke of Jesus and His unfailing love. Of my belonging to Him. Of His heart for the lonely. Of becoming part of God's family.

Belonging. Family.

My spirit instantly knew that this was where I belonged and, more importantly, whom I belonged to. The evangelical speaker did an altar call and my hand shot up. I wanted to know this Jesus. I wanted to belong to Him forever. I didn't care that I had a bad reputation and that most of my peers in the room likely knew that. I just wanted to be healed. With tears streaming down my face, I walked to the front and received a new heart. I kept my journal from that year and I can clearly read how everything changed. The God of Israel began a healing and sanctifying work in me that brisk November night that He is still working on completing today, 22 years later.

Yes, I was transformed instantly. And yes, I was transformed slowly. I'm not sure how those two things go together, but they do. Instantly I knew that premarital sex was off the table, as were all the sins that were clearly outlined in the Bible. I began reading God's Word, a devotional, and *Traveling Light* by Max Lucado. As my high school friend group continued to go out to parties and clubs on weekends, I couldn't wait for extended time to read and be in the presence of the Lord. I loved Him. My Spirit felt the two things it hadn't felt for a very long time, if ever: Safety and home. I focused my energy on getting out of high school. I planned to go to college, study interior design and French, and most importantly, meet my husband so I could begin a family of my own.

BUILDING A FAMILY: TAKE ONE

During my freshman year in college I dated two boys. Two Christian boys. I thought I would marry each and was devastated when, for various reasons, each relationship failed. My desperation grew, and I was no longer trusting the Lord to fill my lonely places; I was looking for a man to do this. I realize now this is called idolatry.

During my sophomore year of college I was working as a teller at a bank and met a man we'll call Motorcycle T. Motorcycle T was not evil, but he was broken, and I still had so much brokenness of my own. Motorcycle T liked me, which was great! I liked him too. He was funny and dangerous. We jumped into a fast and furious relationship and were engaged after three months of dating.

There were a lot of things that Motorcycle T and I did that made life hard for each other after we got married. Brokenness and immaturity are a poor pair. Yet at the ripe age of 22, Motorcycle T gave me the best gift in the entire world. I was going to be a mom!

After ten months and a smooth pregnancy, I stared into the face of a miracle. Tiny nose. Tiny breath. Tiny tears. Head full of black, matted hair. The moment the doctor laid her on my chest in the delivery room, I began a full-blown sermon to the nurses around me declaring the glory of God and His majesty in creating life. I was blown away by God's goodness and mercy. I stared at this tiny being whom I was now 100% responsible for keeping alive, or so it felt. I marveled at how she had been fully formed in my womb whilst I had done nothing more than eat French fries and walk the neighborhood. God. Was. Real.

Motorcycle T and I were thrilled, sleep deprived, still broken, and still trying. With no life raft to hold us afloat, our arguments continued. Only now, we were arguing in front of our precious miracle. This wouldn't do. Eventually we decided in our under-developed-frontal-cortex brains that we would separate for a time to figure out our differences, heal, and provide more peace to the beautiful baby girl we both loved madly.

Separation is rarely the answer to marital struggles, although sometimes it is necessary for safety in extreme circumstances. Our separation did not bring us closer together, it only separated us further. Our two-year-old struggled painfully through this separation. It was devastating. It matched the feelings I had when my own dad left our family. Broken family. Broken heart. Broken. Deeply, irrevocably broken. I had tried for more than ten years to put a family together and had somehow ended up in the exact same place: a shattered heart.

A TIME TO HEAL

This began my single mom years. I was freshly enrolled in graduate school and pursuing a master's degree in psychology when my marriage fell apart. Side note, I would not wish divorce on my worst enemy. God hates divorce because of His deep compassion for us. So there I was–twenty-six and divorced—this was quite possibly my worst nightmare. But the Lord wasn't finished with my story. Not by a long shot.

I got my sweet and spunky toddler to bed early every night and went straight to God's word. I spent a couple of hours before bed reading scripture or devotionals and journaling prayers. I focused my energy on two things: being a good mom and seeking the Lord's healing. Only the One who created my heart could heal it; thankfully I was slowly beginning to realize this.

BUILDING A FAMILY: TAKE TWO

Clinging to God in that season showed me what I needed as opposed to what I wanted; I still wanted a whole and beautiful family of my very own, but I needed God more. So, I sought Him with every ounce of strength I could muster. I've heard it said that love finds us when we stop looking for it. Perhaps there is some truth to this saying. Although I hadn't given up my search completely, I was at least looking to God first.

Enter Matthew. Not the book of the Bible, but a man named Matthew. A tall, single dad from New England, to be exact. I met him one day very serendipitously which is a story for another time. We were friends first. Friendship was followed by a yearlong pure and intentional courtship complete with hand holding, prayers, and studying God's Word. And then came a wedding.

Exhale. Fresh Start. New dreams. Perhaps life could be beautiful once more.

I was twenty-nine and ready to begin building a family again. I had surrendered my heart and life completely to the Lord, followed God's commands of being equally yoked, and I thought the rest would be easy and beautiful. I was ready for my fairytale and couldn't wait to begin growing our family and having more children with the love of my life.

A homestead with lots of kids, laughter, and a farmhouse table . . . Here I come!

INFERTILITY

We got right to work trying for a baby. I felt whole in the area of sexuality, like the Lord had restored the years the locust had eaten.

We had a beautiful union and did things God's way. Three months went by. No baby. Six months later and still no baby. I sensed something was awry, but the doctors told us it could take up to a year and technically we weren't officially infertile until we had been trying for 12 months. Like any sane woman trying to conceive, I spent hours researching what changes I needed to make in my diet. I went into hyperdrive, focusing on our lifestyle choices. I cut out whole food groups. I yelled at my new husband for keeping his cell phone in his pocket as I was sure it was damaging his sperm. I counted, charted, timed, and prayed. One year later, no baby. The following is an excerpt from a blog post I wrote at this point in our journey:

> Many of our friends know our story and have been rooting for us. Matt and I love the Lord with all of our hearts; we desire to serve Him and live redeemed lives. We have both been healed after painful life experiences and the Lord has given us a fresh start together.
>
> With this fresh start, we each have a dream in our hearts to grow our family. I brought a girl to our marriage. Matt brought a boy. Two precious gifts that we love fiercely. And honestly, I pictured us having *at least* 2-3 more children together as being a mom is the greatest joy of my life.
>
> We were so excited and began trying from month one! Six months went by with no pregnancy. Each month I had a reason to think I was pregnant and in this time frame I probably went through at least a hundred pregnancy tests. I had a growing sense that something was wrong, but I was calmly assured that these things take time.

Time. We are often troubled by time. Be it too much, or not enough. We are rushing, or we are having trouble waiting. C.S. Lewis said it like this, "We are so little reconciled to time that we are even astonished at it. 'How he's grown!' we exclaim, 'How time flies!' It's as strange as if a fish were repeatedly surprised at the wetness of water. And that would be strange indeed; unless of course, the fish were destined to become, one day, a land animal" (Lewis, 1958). Yet we have trouble with time because we were not made to live in it. We are made for eternity. Time can be painful and for me, it was. I was wrestling with time. Wrestling with the wait.

For a year, I started each month with the deep hope for that little pink plus sign to show up and ended each month in a puddle of tears. It was time to seek medical help. We saw a primary care physician who ran an analysis. We waited to hear back hoping that this would give us a clue to what we needed to do next. We got more than a clue. The doctor called me a week later—in the middle of my workday—and spoke very matter-of-factly, "You two will probably not have children together. Have you thought about adoption?"

This is not the kind of news you deliver to a woman at three p.m. on a Tuesday afternoon when she's getting ready to sit down with her next client. But he did. I responded in some robotic way, set the phone down, shut my office door, and sobbed harder than I ever had.

I asked God if this was punishment for being divorced. If this was because of all the mistakes I'd made. If He was testing me. I cried out to Him. He was silent.

I went home to tell Matt the news. I tried to maintain my composure, but it was not a pretty night. For several months after that I cried daily and tried to imagine never having a child with my husband. Not a big deal, right? We already have two children. So what if we don't have one together?

I told myself this daily and yet I couldn't let the dream go. My heart ached to grow a family with my husband. To gift these two beautiful children we have with shared siblings. To experience Matt holding my hand in childbirth. To see his gentle-giant hands pick up a tiny life that we've created together. To have this bond with one another that is part of God's purpose for marriage.

We began looking for a second opinion. We met with a fertility specialist who put us on supplements. We tested again three months later, but the outlook was even more bleak. I cried some more. I read a 300-page book on conception and changed each of our diets in drastic ways for six months.

At this point we had been married 21 months. This isn't a long time in the grand scheme of things. Yet twenty-one months of hoping, praying, and crying out to God each month for a blessing you desperately want (but know you don't deserve) was beginning to feel like an eternity.

We went to another specialist who gave us a little more hope, but stated a surgery would be necessary. Thankfully, this specialist found a problem area that others weren't able to locate. After much prayer, we decided to go ahead with the surgery. Neither of us knew what the outcome would be. Although Matt was the one actually having surgery, he was as strong as an oak while I was an emotional wreck.

Struggling with infertility was never part of my formula. It took me by surprise and came at a time when I thought I was leaving the worst of my heartache behind. Life was supposed to now be full of joy and happily-ever-afters. Yet God's plans often look very different from our own. Even in my blog lament, in the midst of struggle, I tried hard to acknowledge that God's ways are higher:

> It's hard to count it all as joy, and yet I'm thankful for a new understanding of what it feels like to face infertility. It gives me another "specialty area" in my counseling ministry, a compassion that is only birthed from experience—but most of all, when and if God decides to give us another child, the glory will be all the more to Him because HE IS ABLE even when doctors say, "not possible." That is the God we serve.

He was able to give us a baby. But that doesn't mean He would. God's will and His ability are two very different things. As I began to lean hard into this truth, I recognized that trust and surrender would become my two best friends.

LETTING GO

More than 21 months went by and then it was three years. After three years, one surgery, countless books on "how to conceive," one visit to an infertility clinic, and a thousand tear-streaked prayers, I let it go. I simply let the dream die. Like a balloon floating up to the sky, I watched the dream drift further and further away from my life. I tried to imagine life without this dream.

Perhaps it's more honest to say that the balloon string was pried from my white-knuckled grip. I had tried to force God's will to align with mine, but life doesn't work that way. The dream had to float away if my hands were going to be open to hold what was in front of me. I couldn't love what was in my life by desperately scheming to get what wasn't there. I finally realized that having a baby was not within my locus of control. It didn't matter what I did or how hard I tried, this was a decision that was up to God, and I had to give it to Him. Completely. I cried and grieved. I asked *why* and then I gave Him the balloon.

As it goes, when my heart was completely prostrated before Jesus and I was broken to the point of surrender, God decided to give the dream back, in His way and His timing. I was scheduled and way overdue for wisdom teeth extraction and out of an abundance of caution, I decided to take *just one more* pregnancy test before heading to the oral surgeon's office. Surprise! It was a plus sign. I took another test. Another plus sign. In disbelief, my hands trembled. One more pregnancy test—another plus sign. Could it be that after years of wrestling with God, then surrendering and giving the dream to Him, that He was giving it back?

SELAH: PAUSE, PONDER, AND PRAY

The months that followed were a joyful and blurred frenzy. Matt and I barely hit the 8-week mark before we began telling friends and strangers alike. We went out to celebrate and posted on social media.

We declared the goodness of God! Our long-awaited child was on the way! Our kids, family members, and friends were thrilled for us.

Like every woman with access to Pinterest, we planned a reveal party with family. This was planned for the very day that I had my ultrasound to find out the baby's gender. I would have my appointment at two p.m., come home to get the house ready, and guests would arrive at five.

I never for one second considered that our baby might not be healthy. The thought never crossed my mind. We had waited three long years, prayed without ceasing, and now God had been gracious; a healthy baby was on the way. Or so I thought. During the ultrasound, the tech was quiet. Too quiet. She ran the machine over my belly again and again and then quietly walked us back to meet with the doctor. My heart felt heavy. What did all this quiet noise mean?

It is clear in my mind still today. The doctor walked in and said, "Your baby is a girl, but she's very sick." No amount of preparation can prepare a mother for those words. She went on to explain that the baby's kidneys had cysts, her bladder had a cyst, and that we would need to meet with a specialist right away. The room was spinning, and I was spouting questions about what I needed to do.

The doctor placed her hand on my knee, looked me gently in the eyes and said, "I know if there was anything you could do, you would do it because that's the type of mother you are. But there's nothing you can do. We just need to see what we're dealing with."

I was hot and cold at the same time. I was alone in a crowded room. I looked at Matt. Our scared eyes found one another's and he grabbed my hand. There were no words. Our long awaited, long prayed-for child was on the way, and she was sick. The formal diagnosis was either MCDK or PCDK (multicystic or polycystic kidneys), and whichever diagnosis this sweet new baby had would determine if she would live or not. MCDK babies can sometimes fare okay, while polycystic kidneys cannot support life.

I went home. We had our gender reveal party and shared a sugar-coated version of the news, "It's a girl! She may have some kidney issues, so please pray." I was a robot through that night. I was in denial; I couldn't even speak the words to close family members that our baby was sick.

The following months consisted of weekly appointments with our specialist and weekly ultrasounds to monitor the baby and the amount of amniotic fluid in my womb. Plans were made to deliver early in case of dropping amniotic fluid levels. I was trying desperately to get to the 30-week mark with her . . . and then 32 weeks . . . and then 34. In two-week increments and three a.m. ugly-cry prayers, we made it through the second half of pregnancy.

Around the 32nd week, we were told at the specialist's office that a major brain structure was missing. It was a gut punch. It was Christmas time, and I was in church a lot singing Christmas songs on our church worship team and thinking about how Mary felt bringing her baby into the world. Thinking about her fear of all the unknowns. How she must have been utterly bewildered by the events of her young life, and yet had found grace and peace. If Jesus is all He says He is, then live or die, my baby would live with Him, and I would meet her one day. I tried to wrap my human mind around this eternal truth for comfort.

As I prayed for the new life forming in my womb, a name seemed to bubble up from within me. It was as if my baby already had a name, and I was trying to hear clearly what it was. *Stella? Was it Stella? No, that wasn't right.* I couldn't make out the name, yet it was there in my prayers. Then one morning during a sermon, our pastor said the word "Selah" and as soon as I heard it, I knew that was the name of our baby girl. It was her God-given name and I didn't choose it, I only recognized it. "Selah" means to pause, ponder, and praise—and amidst all the heartache and waiting and unknowns of those final months, I would choose to do just that.

Christmas came slowly and I chose to be present, to pause, and ponder. If God had already given me a living daughter and had answered years of cries to create a new life with my husband, couldn't He also make her live? Indeed, He could, but would He? I didn't know, yet

I had to trust His character. I had to trust that He knew best. So, we prayed and asked everyone we knew to pray. Pray. Trust. Wait.

We made it through Christmas and into January. At 34 weeks, my amniotic fluid began to get low, which meant the baby's kidneys weren't producing enough fluid. We picked a date for induction. The following week the fluid levels were low but stable, so we pushed the plan out just a little more, trying to get the baby to the 36-week marker.

Day by day, we somehow made it to 36 weeks. We were told by the medical team that we couldn't risk waiting any longer to deliver the baby so she could be monitored in the hospital. We were also prepared for stillbirth. There were so many unknowns. The morning of February 6th, we got up at six a.m. and were at the hospital by seven. Matt and I played Yahtzee as they began to pump my veins with Pitocin to get labor started. I read Psalm 23. We held hands. We played more Yahtzee. By three in the afternoon things weren't progressing, so they broke my water.

Things got intense after that and by seven that night our baby girl was here. Many doctors and specialists visited us. They poked her, drew blood, scanned her kidneys, but always brought her right back to me. They frantically demanded I nurse her more. I tried. She wasn't getting enough fluid.

On day three of our baby's life, day three in our dark hospital room surrounded by beeping monitors and cords, Selah took a turn for the better. My milk came in and scans showed—miracle of miracles— only one kidney had cysts. We only needed her to have one function- ing kidney, so this meant that she would live!

She would LIVE. On day three, she would LIVE. Just like Jesus on the third day rose from his tomb back to life, this dream which had died several times over in my mind and heart over the last three years came to life and LIVED.

Selah.

Her big sister, Brooke, couldn't come to the hospital to meet her due to restrictions, but I'll never forget the day Brooke first saw her long-awaited little sister. Brooke was eight years old, and her faith became real that day. She saw that after her own eternity of longing and praying for a sister, God answered. Malakai was 13 and Selah quickly earned a place in big brother's heart as she gazed at him with her miracle-eyes. The four of us welcomed our new family member home. Joy froze time. We were a family of five. We were a family.

LIFE TODAY

As I write today, Selah is now five years old. And guess what? When Selah was six months old, we became surprise pregnant with another baby! Our surprise baby boy, Ari, is four. "Ari" means *lion of God.* He is snuggly and kind and covered in dark hair–a true man-child. He rushed down the birth canal and into this world at 9 pounds, 11 ounces. He loves trucks, mama, and his big, wild family. The fact that God poured out His mercy in the form of a double blessing still leaves me speechless.

This broken girl from a broken home with broken and dead dreams now writes to you as a mom of four. Matt and I just finished raising our eldest son, who turned 18, asked to get baptized, and then joined the Marines earlier this year. We are still working on raising a stunning, creative, and hilarious 14-year-old daughter, a 6-year-old with a laugh that lights up a room, and a 4-year-old whose snuggles could melt an ice queen.

Four kids. God gave this lonely, fatherless, divorced, and broken girl a godly husband and four kids. For He is truly "A father to the fatherless, a defender of widows, is God in His holy dwelling. God sets the lonely in families" (Psalm 68:5-6a, NIV).

Building a family didn't go as I had planned. My attempts to form it myself only led to more heartache. It was only a fully surrendered heart and open hands that allowed me to grasp the dream God was and still is building today. To be clear, life is not a fairy-tale; it is hard in many ways. Hard and beautiful. Selah still sees specialists at hospitals all over our state. She can't eat certain foods, take ibuprofen, or play contact sports because she has only one kidney. She may need medical intervention when she gets older. Indeed, all of our days are numbered. Yet she is a living, breathing, constant reminder to pause, ponder, and praise.

Nothing was ever in my control, but miracles abound in all four of our miracle babes. May I—and may we—never forget that life is full of miracles.

"'For this child I prayed, and the Lord has granted me my petition, which I asked of Him. Therefore I also have lent him to the Lord; as long as he lives he shall be lent to the Lord.' So they worshiped the Lord there." (1 Samuel 1: 27-28. NKJV)

REFERENCES

Lewis, C.S. *Reflections on the Psalms*. (1958). San Diego: Harcourt, Brace and Company.

CHAPTER SIX

IMMEASURABLY MORE

By Karen Campbell

Thought I would see you moving by now,
but I don't see you moving.
Thought that you would be here by now,
but I don't see you coming.
I am supposed to seek you and find you
but I feel like you're hiding.
Where do I go with my dreams?
Where do I go with this longing?
Thought you would come this way, to heal this broken heart.
My spirit is broken, you took everything I submitted
to your will, but I am still left hoping.
What am I to do?
Where am I to go?
I thought I had it figured out. But now I just don't know.
You keep me waiting, ever anticipating.
My longing unending, my soul breaking and bending.
Lord, I need you to come.
—K. Campbell

Our parenthood story begins two years into our marriage with three tender words: "There's no heartbeat." My wide-eyed 24-year-old face fell flat. My husband Bryan held my hand. I knew in that dimly lit examination room that the moment was too big for me. The mountain was too high. I felt too young to be experiencing something so grown up. In a matter of weeks I had to reconcile rejoicing in the idea of becoming a mother with this new journey of grief. I know that I wasn't listening when the nurse gave me a list of instructions and I walked out of the room only to be greeted with expecting mothers in the waiting room. I didn't even know how to move forward and I had no language for my feelings. I had never experienced such a beautiful beginning with such a heartbreaking ending. With the help of family and friends I learned what it meant to grieve, but it felt like we had to grow up quickly with this heartache.

I missed our baby more times than I let on. I got good at hiding my pain and would smile my way through the day. I could talk in circles about how I was okay so that no one would know the complete shock and sadness that lingered in my heart. Baby gifts that we had received were put out of sight, and I was confused as to why the Lord allowed it. After our miscarriage we tried to celebrate the fourth of July. The fireworks were so brightly lit across the sky. With every boom of the firework display, I found myself turning inward. I hoped I could move forward with grace, but I didn't know how. I learned how to push through, to say I was good, but the longing in my heart wouldn't leave. And it never did. We gave ourselves a year for our hearts to heal but I never felt that I was the same person after losing our baby at 12 weeks. I was different. I had different dreams and my heart became tenderer to the miracle of life.

Then the Lord put the desire in our hearts to try again to build our family. I'm glad I didn't know at the time that it would take us almost five years to become pregnant. With endless doctor visits, it felt like time was not on our side. We were told everything from, "relax, it will happen," to "it may never happen." The road of infertility was daunting, unpredictable, and often lonely. I remember reaching for my husband's hand and crying myself to sleep many nights. I threw myself into graduate school to distract myself and found a love of learning. Graduate school made me happy, and some joy returned to my life. I also traveled and participated in overseas missions but still dreamed of becoming a mother.

As the years went by and my aching heart tried to hold on to hope, we sought the advice of fertility specialists who often spoke with confusing statistics. I was frustrated sitting in one office after another trying to find answers. I was determined, even stubborn, in my pursuit of information that could help us. Bryan often caught me dozing off while reading books on infertility. I remember having to endure painful Mother's Day church services every year so I started to avoid them. I didn't want to be told that my biggest calling in life was motherhood. I wanted more. I wanted God. I had always thought my relationship with the Lord was strong but I was faced with the fact that He was not giving us the desire of our hearts. He didn't seem to be answering my prayers, so I finally had to ask the questions: Would I trust Him when my hands were empty? Would I move forward with Him if that meant never becoming a mother? I had to wrestle with all of this. I remembered Colossians 1:17, "He is before all things, and in Him all things hold together" which was spoken over our marriage years before. I clung to this truth. No matter the outcome, I believed Christ was holding us together as we waited and prayed for our family to grow.

During this challenging journey I felt the Lord speak to me in a number of ways. While shopping one day, I came across a small sign with one simple word, HOPE, and I knew at that moment, hope was all that I had. I had hope in the Lord. I had hope in His Word and hope that he was hearing my cries. But more than anything, I knew I had my relationship with Christ. It sustained me (Isaiah 46:4). I knew the sign was for me and I purchased it. I put it in my home, passed by it daily, and pondered the word. God's hope infused my soul and I knew that He could "do immeasurably more than all we ask or imagine, according to His power that is at work within us" (Ephesians 3:20).

That verse followed me across the ocean as I ministered to children overseas. God encouraged me to put all my hope in Him and to expect miracles. My faith began to grow and I welcomed my pastor's wife and my close friend to hold onto hope with me. I was not hoping alone. If this heartache was going to be a part of my journey, I knew I needed to whisper my greatest fears to my most trusted friends.

After another long year of trying, my husband and I took a trip to the beach alone. We felt exhausted and just needed time away. I knew there was a chance that I could take a pregnancy test on this trip but I was also hoping to focus just on rest. I remember waking up one morning and deciding not to wait any longer. I walked into the bathroom and took what felt like my 100th pregnancy test and before I could even blink I saw two pink lines staring back at me. I was shocked. I literally shook as I shared the news with my sweet husband who was beyond excited. We celebrated and I felt that hope rising up in my heart again. We planned and prayed and rejoiced with friends as we found out we were having a son. It was a blessed time and one I will never forget. Our beloved son Caleb was on his way and we named him after the story in the Bible about how Caleb believed when others didn't. Caleb means faithful and we knew that our God was.

Caleb came abruptly into the world five weeks early. I held our adorable baby boy in my arms and declared John 16:33 over him "I have told you these things, so that in me you may have peace. In this world you will have trouble. But take heart! I have overcome the world." I whispered to him that he was an overcomer. I wanted to be strong at that moment but I wept when they took him out of my arms and rushed him to the NICU. It was one of the hardest moments of my life.

We prayed for Caleb and family and friends came in shifts to the hospital. During that time, the only face that brought me relief was my husband's. He was the main person that endured with me the painful story of infertility and grief. It seemed we were ushered into a new story of even greater uncertainty. He was the one who knew how we both longed and waited to look into Caleb's beautiful blue eyes. To have

Caleb swiftly whisked away was like an echo of the road we thought we had left. Caleb wouldn't stay awake long enough to eat and although the doctors meant well, they had more questions than answers. We didn't rest for almost two weeks but by God's grace we were able to take Caleb home with precautions. This letting go of control and trusting the Lord to guide us became our new normal.

We went home and threw ourselves into caring for our son around the clock like most parents do. He was behind in weight and we had to intently monitor his milk intake. That job easily took two people. My husband and I worked in shifts and before long we were utterly exhausted, but Caleb made us so happy and was such a joy to hold and snuggle. We prayed that God would heal him and we asked our loving church family to help us. Weeks flew by and at his four-month check-up his doctor noted some concerns. Even in the uncertainty, I knew that holding my son was nothing short of a miracle. God's miracle.

My nights and days were turned upside down as I started to understand that my son had physical delays that were going unexplained. I had postpartum anxiety that seemed to linger. Caleb's life was such a gift but my heart was heavy with the weight of being a new mother. Caleb wouldn't eat. We lost sleep. Developmental milestones were not reached. My nights were filled with insomnia and nightmares; my husband would find me awake sitting with my arms open. "What are you doing? " he asked. "I'm catching Caleb," I said in my sleep-deprived state. The nightmare of my son falling toward me with my arms wide open happened several nights in a row. "I have you buddy, we got you." I'd say. *But who had me? Who had my marriage?* These intrusive thoughts met me every night and my deepest inadequacies met me every morning. I was not living up to who I thought I was and shame sat with me like a wounded friend. The worry, anxiety, and sleepless nights began to take its toll and I found myself in a spiritual wilderness. As I felt myself losing hope, I wept for the Lord not to lose hold of me. I remember speaking directly to one of my sisters during those long weeks and she dropped everything to come be with me. I could see with help and direction that I had to start living differently and purposely as I fought to stay afloat in this new season.

Over time, I started to speak more kindly to myself and started to gently create new rhythms in our home. I was grieving these unreached milestones for my son and our family and needed space to do so. I let go of my career and Caleb and I learned and laughed together. His zest for life became my joy. Caleb grew and I no longer wanted out of my story but to step into this new life of learning what my son needed. Appointments and therapies filled our weeks.

During this season of new rhythms, we were blessed with another pregnancy! Our first daughter was to be born and we were elated with God's kindness. I began to pray scripture over Caleb, and over our new baby daughter, Kate, when she arrived. Every day I prayed Psalm 23:6 over them, that goodness and mercy would follow them all the days of their lives. I sang praise songs to push back my fears and doubts of parenting two children and also waiting on a diagnosis for Caleb. I declared Psalm 16:8 over my marriage, that with God, we would not be shaken. I was hungry for God and believed Matthew 5:6, "Blessed are those who hunger and thirst for righteousness, for they shall be satisfied." Soon after Kate turned one we were delighted to find out we were pregnant with our third child, Allyson. God was doing more than we could ask or imagine right in front of our eyes. We smiled and rejoiced over all three of them.

During this season we also got more answers as we found out that Caleb had a rare myopathy, and we began to piece together what he needed to thrive. Each day offered me a new perspective to see the story God was writing. I let my heart break wide open for God to teach me to be the mother I needed to be. I began to work diligently to make our home our safe place and to nurture them with the love of God. Delighting in our three miracles became a deep joy in my life. I embraced this breathtaking freedom: That God orchestrates our lives. This new lived out truth helped me move forward. My husband's leadership and friendship had always been dear to me but it started to become even clearer to me that we were meant for this journey together. I began to see that opening up my hands freed me to love the people in my life well.

Caleb is 12 now and is becoming a caring young man. He is incredibly fast in his wheelchair and at times, I can't even catch him. His quick wit, kindness, creativity, and love for learning have made me love life more. He is the son I always wanted. My daughters are the lifelong friends my heart longed for. Each one of our children is teaching me something about my faith and about the Lord's love. I couldn't have dreamed up their personalities or gifts and it all feels like a love letter from my Father in heaven when I think about how much we prayed for them. Our family and friends have been so supportive and we couldn't have made it this far without them. We are grateful for their love.

All three of our children are miracles. They are the miracles we longed for, prayed for, and are miracles we didn't deserve. When I see our children talking, laughing, and growing, I am in awe of what God has done. I have been able to see God more clearly and know that He is not distant but present. I am someone who wrestled with her faith and watched God move mountains. In Galatians 5:6 it states that what counts is faith expressing itself through love. I am praying that my family demonstrates this kind of faith to each other and those in our lives. My purpose is to know the Lord and say *yes* to Him in faith. To give Him my dreams. And remember that hope sign? That hope sign now sits in my office as I remember what the Lord has done and proclaim his goodness. It's my Ebenezer. I'll always remember how God took my brokenness and brought forth new life. Thanks be to God.

CHAPTER SEVEN

YOUR DREAMS AREN'T BIG ENOUGH

By Laura Davis

I met the man who would be my handsome golden-haired, blue-eyed husband, Timothy, on the day I moved into my college apartment. Stepping through my apartment's front door with his younger brother (who was dating my roommate) was the perfect opportunity to ask this good-looking guy for help. A few months later we attempted to study together on a warm Sunday afternoon at a country lake but found ourselves in delightful summer crush bliss. This gentleman of a man compassionately put others first and I fell deep in love. Conversations of a future together and dreams of starting a family followed. Many dates later he dropped to one knee on the sandy west coast Florida shore and asked for my hand in marriage. After eighteen months of dating, we tied the knot on an unusually warm winter day.

Playing "Mommy" came naturally to me since I was a little girl and my biggest dream was to become a mom. Barefoot and pregnant in my early 20s sounded perfect to me. But, as many couples do, we decided to wait three to five years until we could afford more than spaghetti for dinner every night.

A few years into our marriage my husband swept me off my feet and booked a romantic bed and breakfast out of town to begin our long-awaited dream of having children. No one can truly describe the secret joy a husband and wife share when they are hoping for a little bundle of love to rock in their arms.

Month after month, we waited for our ship to come in, but it never arrived at our dock. We decided to pursue medical testing. I'll never forget the day I came home to red roses on our kitchen counter and a note. Zero percent chance. Radiation from childhood leukemia stole the dream tucked away in both our hearts that we never knew we'd have to relinquish. Prior to the roses that day, on a long bike ride, my husband and God hashed out the grief of that lost dream. It took me years to work through my grief. I know that we certainly can take steps to improve the chances of a miracle, but ultimately it is fully in the hands of Christ. Even if it looked differently than we imagined.

I felt immense joy to finally have a plan for building our family through adoption yet at the same time, I mourned the death of a baby-carrying dream I never knew I'd bury. Prayers were prayed, natural method books read, healthy diets tried, words of comfort offered. No baby bump came. No announcements were squealed. No maternity dresses worn. Time stood still in our inability to get pregnant. Yet, since the initial knowledge of pregnancy complication possibilities, we had already decided in vitro fertilization interventions were not a path we wanted to take.

After much prayer, conversations with adoptive families, and re-searching adoption agencies, we created a profile for a local birthmother. My heart ached for her to choose us as adoptive parents for the little one in her womb. Then plans and places changed. Within a week we completed the paperwork to initiate an adoption from Taiwan. Fortunately, God stopped us in our tracks in order to show us the need in Congo, Africa. My sister-in-law showed me pictures from a blog of a woman who had adopted from Congo and my heart broke. The pictures showed a dark room, one toy for too many children, and contaminated water.

I was done. I talked with Tim and he was on board to do whatever God called us to do even though we knew that an adoption from Congo would be more risky, expensive, and unsafe. On my knees on our bathroom floor I can remember praying, "Lord, even if we don't adopt from Congo, LORD, will you please provide for these children." God responded, " No Laura, YOU will provide for these children."

After endless hours of paperwork, multiple background checks, adoption education training, vaccinations, a home inspection, adoptive parent questionnaires, prayers, tears, waiting, and more waiting, it was finally time. Three airplanes and one van ride down a dirt road filled with potholes, and we were there. The place where we met our little one. We were terrified and excited. On that summer day we met our beautiful Congolese daughter who still captivates our hearts. You see, we planned to adopt a baby, but God planned something much better. He found a way to intervene in two tragic situations to create mysterious beauty. Our daughter forever changed our hearts.

When you consider the grief, tragedy, and change an orphan endures, it makes sense that such a delicate little life can challenge you. It was a difficult but beautiful time in our home as we adjusted to becoming a family. Our new daughter learned to trust us and know that we'd never leave. We learned God's relentless love for us. We clearly understood how God adopted us as orphans, taking us into His family to be forever loved. I came to understand passages like Galatians 4:3-7: "In the same way we also, when we were children, were enslaved to the elementary principles of this world. But when the fullness of time had come, God sent forth his Son, born of woman, born under the law, to redeem those who were under the law, so that we might receive adoption as sons. And because you are sons, God has sent the Spirit of his Son into our hearts, crying, "Abba! Father!" So you are no longer a slave, but a son, and if a son, an heir through God." We also clung to Ephesians 1:5: "He predestined us for adoption to himself as sons through Jesus Christ, according to the purpose of his will, to the praise of his glorious grace, with which he has blessed us in the Beloved."

We became a tight-knit family of three yet knew in our hearts that we didn't want our family to stop at that number. Our next attempt at adopting went from what we thought would be two years to seven long years of waiting, hoping, excitement, and loss. Some families' adoption stories from start to finish are only nine months (true story–this is how long it took my husband's brother and his wife to adopt our adorable little nephew from Korea). Every family has its own story timeline, and we all have expectations: college, marriage, house, and baby. You know what I'm talking about. Those are timelines we mistakenly make without asking God what HIS timeline is for our life. God's timing is absolutely impeccable and I don't know why it took me so long to surrender our "life timelines" to Him.

In short, we tried to adopt a little boy from Congo. However, the doors closed because of red tape. We were approached about adopting twins from Tanzania. The doors closed again. So we became foster parents and were asked to adopt twin baby boys. That door closed after we had already prepared their room. We heard of the opportunity to adopt that little boy from Congo again, along with a little girl this time. We prayed so hard and our adoption agency was willing to bend over backwards to try to make a way when there wasn't one. The situation was extremely risky and the possibility of success was very low. Needless to say, in a period of waiting for six years, we "lost" six children. I felt like I had "miscarried" six times.

In all the years we searched for who would join our family, I never realized how loud my voice was. Tim had introduced the idea of Haiti at the beginning of our adoption journey but my mama bear aching heart had dismissed the notion, thinking it would take "way too long." Well, let's just say that perhaps I didn't have a clue. Little did I know that God would prompt my heart for where our first little one would come from, and then, for our second adoption, prompt Tim's.

We stepped into the Haitian adoption process ready to fill out every form and get the ball rolling. The program was well run and we were on our way to adopt our next little one. On a warm summer day with homemade bread in the oven and while cleaning our blinds (two things I rarely do) I got THE call. "Would you consider adopting twins?" The agency could share little information at the time but asked if we would be willing to be one of the families, amongst others, who could adopt these little ones. Almost one year later we received another call that we were CHOSEN! This time, our oldest daughter would join us on our journey to bring home her new little brother and sister.

Life ended up looking way different than I'd ever pictured in my mind. Yet, the picture created by Our Creator is WAY better than what I could have drawn with my few dull crayons. Three children, seven years apart, sounds crazy to me. But you know what? I look into those faces every day and I LOVE them. Our little "Peanut's" (lil sis) prayers can move mountains. Little man is hilarious. Coconut baby (our first) will challenge you to see Christ as He really is. She's an incredible big sis.

We learned so many lessons. The first is that when we let go of a dream we've held onto and get on board with what God wants to do, more lives are changed. The death of one dream makes room for the birth of a new one. Don't hold onto a dream that's not happening for you and miss out on lives waiting to be changed. It's okay to not have all the answers when people ask. God has the answers.

We also learned that it's okay to not share every detail of your children's orphan stories. The grief of an adopted child is excruciatingly painful no matter how old the child is. As much as you want to heal this hurt, you can't, only God can. Sometimes just sitting in the mess of tear-stained faces of grief is better comfort than any words.

I've learned it's okay to ask for pickles and ice cream even if you're not pregnant. A good husband will still get them for you. Can I also just say that it's not okay for random, well-meaning people to ask if we can't get pregnant? I mean, come on, when have I ever asked you about your sex life?

Another lesson is that your own fear may be standing in the way of releasing someone from a life of little hope. Pastor Brad Lotz of Hill City Church once said something in a sermon that has always stuck with me: "Do it scared." DO the thing God's calling you to do, even if it scares the living daylights out of you. An absolutely incredible adoption and foster resource called *The Orphan Care Advocacy Organization Archibald Project* urges people: "Don't let the desire to be comfortable stand in the way of something you're called to do."

The first verse I ever memorized after accepting Christ as my Savior was Psalm 37:4, which says "Delight yourself in the Lord and HE will give you the desires of your heart." That verse stood out to me at the time because I thought it meant that if I followed Christ, my dreams would come true. Little did I know the accurate meaning was the more I learned and pursued God's heart by reading the Bible, praying, and seeking to honor Him with my choices, that HE would put HIS desires in my heart.

Thank you, God, that YOUR dreams for me were much greater than mine. I'm honored to be the mommy of our three. Our next calling is to grow our family again. When we were foster parents for a short season, God placed a calling on our lives to foster teens. That season is around the corner and we've begun preparing for what's next. My most recent prayer has echoed from a simple yet brilliant prayer in Justin Whitmel Earley's book *Habits of the Household: Practicing the Story of God in Everyday Rhythms*, "Parent us, so we can parent our children."[1] My prayer is the same for you.

REFERENCES

Earley, J. W. (2021) *Habits of the household: Practicing the story of God in everyday family rhythms.* Grand Rapids, MI: Zondervan.

CHAPTER EIGHT

PURPLE FLOWER

By Kristina Lace

Surprise and panic gripped me as I glanced down at my cell phone while driving to work at 7:20 am. My OBGYN's phone number was on the screen. Confusion and fear overwhelmed me as the pit of my stomach dropped. Kelley, my husband, had had a semen analysis done the day before, but why in the world would the doctor call so early? I'd never had a call at this hour before. I stared at the phone in a moment of paralysis, assuming the worst. In my experience, early morning or late-night calls usually weren't good ones.

I answered the call with one hand on the wheel and my eyes fixated on the road before me. It was the first time I had ever heard such a concerned tone coming from a doctor, and it grabbed my complete attention in the most alarming way. He explained that the results of Kelley's semen analysis were not good. In fact, he said they were some of the most concerning results he'd ever seen and he recommended Kelley see an urologist immediately. My legs went numb and my mind began to race with this new information. So many questions began to swirl in my head. *Was there something life-threateningly wrong with my husband? If so, would he be okay? Would we ever be able to have biological children?*

The doctor knew the news was extremely heavy and he attempted to comfort me; that's when I lost control and began to cry. Through my voice cracking I managed to get out the questions, "Do you think he's okay? Will we be able to have kids?" He paused, and that pause conveyed all I needed to know. He didn't even have to answer my questions. His silent doubt cut like a razor. He chose his response carefully in order to be sensitive. He didn't want to give me false hope, yet he wanted to comfort me. He simply replied, "I'm not sure. I hope so, but I'm just not sure." With that phone call my husband and I entered uncharted territory and began a journey that changed us forever. We had no idea what lay ahead. My doctor's hope in that moment, as small as it sounded, was what I clung to. It was the first of many times that I had to desperately hold onto hope when things looked hopeless.

I'm sharing our infertility story with its rollercoaster ride of emotions and seemingly insurmountable struggles to help remove some of the stigma and shame for those who experience a difficult path to parenthood. It is my prayer that our story can be a source of hope and help to normalize the internal and external battles of infertility. It's the story of how we kept following God, seeking answers, and made it through by grace. Professor and author Brene Brown said that the two most powerful words when we're struggling are "me too." (Brown, 2012). That "me too" feeling, the one where we feel less alone, can be powerful and healing for us. My biggest hope in sharing all of this with you is that you'll connect with something in our story and think, "me too" and you'll feel less alone.

I grew up on a small dairy farm in southwest Missouri where I was surrounded by nature, livestock, and pets. Some of my earliest memories include dressing up a few chosen farm-cats-turned-pets in doll clothes and treating them like my babies. Fur babies, but you get the point. From the early age of seven I knew I wanted to be a mom. It was definitely an instinct built into me and something I both wanted and expected.

After high school, I decided to pursue a career that rivals farming as far as hard work is concerned: Teaching. I was halfway through my degree when I met my husband, Kelley, on a church ski trip. He literally skied backwards down a hill to teach me how to ski, was incredibly patient, and pretty cute and funny, too. We married and I got my first teaching job shortly after as a fourth-grade teacher. I had previously worked at the after school and summer daycare programs through the same school district and was thrilled to be teaching some of the students I already knew and loved like crazy.

After about three years of marriage, Kelley and I decided to try to build our family. It was all part of the equation, right? Boy meets girl, they marry, and then have a baby. We were both so excited to be parents, so of course, I started planning. As a teacher who planned things down to the minute, I had already determined when I needed to get pregnant in order to have my maternity leave over summer break. I shared our plan with my OBGYN and during our initial discussion my husband's family history of cystic fibrosis seemed to cause him a bit of concern. However, he continued and advised us to try for a year as most couples conceive within this time. I had no reason to believe we wouldn't be one of those couples. However, after trying for only nine months I felt in my gut something might be wrong. My mom and sister had each conceived within three months so I had a nagging feeling something was off. Plus, to be honest, my impatience kicked in as well. *We were both young, healthy, and doing everything in our power to get pregnant, so why wasn't it working?* I called my doctor and his first step was to schedule a semen analysis for Kelley because I'd already had baseline fertility tests, which were normal.

Fast forward to the early morning call that changed our family-building plans. After the call, Kelley was referred to a local urologist within the week, which was a sign of the severity of the diagnosis. The urologist shared that he didn't believe there was anything life-threatening such as cancer but diagnosed Kelley with azoospermia due to unilateral absence of vas deferens. Basically, due to his family history of cystic fibrosis, he was born with a blockage that prevented his sperm from getting where it needed to go and it was severely impacting his sperm count. It's similar to a vasectomy except he was born with the condition. The urologist explained that if we wanted to pursue having biological children, we'd need to meet with a reproductive endocrinologist–an infertility specialist. Because there were none in Southwest Missouri we would have the choice of traveling to either Kansas City or St. Louis. I had a teacher friend who was receiving treatment at a clinic in Kansas City, so due to that personal connection, I chose KC. In hindsight, I didn't do any research about the clinic as it pertained to its expertise in male factor fertility, which might have been unwise. If I had done more research, perhaps we wouldn't have gone there and faced as much adversity. However, I also recognize that God used our entire journey full of struggles, pain, loss, and grief to not only stretch our faith but to also teach us in the process.

During my childhood I watched my mom advocate for my brother who battled epilepsy and she fought for his health in many ways. As we prepared for our appointment in Kansas City, I had no idea how her persevering example would be important to me in our journey. I knew I had enough fight and desire in my heart to be a mom and wasn't going to give up easily. I knew we'd be parents eventually; I just wasn't sure of the path. I was discouraged but held onto hope and was ready for what was ahead. We prayed, had family and close friends pray, and we got busy.

One of the first tests we took was a cystic fibrosis genetic test to see if we were carriers of the gene. I tested negative while Kelley tested positive. Kelley's uncle had cystic fibrosis and passed away at the age of 17, so the news that Kelley was a carrier was not completely surprising. The doctor believed this gene had compromised the full formation of his vas deferens, which is the tube that transports sperm. Because of this Kelley would require a special procedure to extract viable sperm. The doctor also diagnosed me with Polycystic Ovary Syndrome (PCOS) and prescribed a drug called Metformin, which is typically given to diabetic patients to lower their blood sugar. I remember secretly questioning the PCOS diagnosis because I had regular periods, ovulated monthly, and was not overweight. I was much younger at the time and didn't push back on the diagnosis. I simply trusted he knew what was best. Even when a side effect of Metformin gave me extreme stomach pain, I still pushed on because I wanted to make sure I was doing everything I could to help our chances of getting pregnant.

We were placed on the fast track to in vitro fertilization (IVF) due to Kelley's diagnosis and started to look at an IVF schedule and a financial plan. This particular clinic participated in a shared risk program, which guaranteed we'd get 80% of our money back if we didn't have a live birth. At the time, it seemed like the best option, so that's what we planned. The financial amount required was shocking and would not be covered by insurance (I strongly believe it should be), but we didn't hesitate to take out a loan for the chance to become parents. This was unfair in our eyes but since parenthood was our most important dream, it was a no-brainer. We scheduled our first fresh IVF cycle, and the protocol included birth control pills, Lupron shots, gonal-f shots (which grew the ovarian follicles into mature eggs for retrieval), a "trigger shot" that signaled my body to release the eggs, and progesterone shots. Estrogen patches were in there somewhere too. It was information overload to say the least. It was definitely a lot to endure, but the physical part was surprisingly not too intimidating for me. Much like the work ethic I'd learned on the farm and through my education, I knew it was what I had to do to reach our goal. I definitely had enough grit for that part of it. However, it was the emotional and spiritual parts that followed that tested my patience, identity, mental health, and faith.

I can still remember the excitement and pride I felt when I saw the flutter of the heartbeat of our seven-week-old fetus on the ultrasound screen. The first cycle had resulted in a pregnancy and we were told by the ultrasound tech that only five percent of women miscarry after seeing the heartbeat. I'm not sure if that statistic was accurate, but if it was, at our 12-week checkup with our OBGYN we learned that we were sadly part of that five percent. I distinctly remember the doctor's words,

"I'm sorry, but there's no heartbeat." He moved us into his office where he kindly explained next steps, prayed for us, and sent us on our way. In a daze, we left the office and cried in devastation when we reached the car. I went from the high of being pregnant to the nightmarish hell of losing a baby we desperately prayed for, worked for, and wanted so much. My doctor also suggested a D&C since my body didn't recognize the miscarriage. It seemed my body was failing me again. Two hits, one after another. I didn't want to be alone, often woke up in the middle of the night sobbing, and eventually had to take sleeping pills to get through that time of loss and grief. It was horrific. Not only had our unborn baby died but we also faced the reality of not knowing if we'd be able to get pregnant again. Thankfully, we had an incredible support system of family, friends, and coworkers who helped, encouraged, and prayed for us during that time. They were vital during our recovery.

As soon as I had the physical clearance from the doctor we decided to try again. We were still hopeful and wanted to continue as soon as possible. We did a frozen cycle (one remaining embryo from the first fresh cycle) and two more fresh cycles for a total of four IVF cycles. Because only three mature eggs made it to the day five transfer date in the first cycle the doctor increased the amount of ovarian stimulating drugs for the following two fresh cycles. Even with the dosage increase, my body was not cooperating and doing quite the opposite–producing hardly any eggs at all. It was the complete opposite effect the doctor had expected. Because of the poor ovarian responses, my doctor added another diagnosis to my file: DOV or Diminished Ovarian Reserve. I was in disbelief. I was only 27 years old and had always had normal menstrual cycles. I couldn't wrap my mind around the diagnosis and neither could my parents. I remember my dad, in particular, being concerned about the amount of medication I was taking. As a farmer, his experience with cattle had taught him to be mindful of weight versus dosage. He told me, in a joking yet serious way, that I needed to gain more weight because he thought the doctor might be prescribing too much medicine. I found it funny that he was comparing me to one of his cows, but I understood the concept and his concern. It was another moment of pause for me. I was already making myself sick on Metformin due to a questionable PCOS diagnosis and now the idea that the doctor might have it wrong with my medication dosage and DOV diagnosis had me questioning our care altogether.

As it turned out, our doctor retired shortly after the 4th cycle (3 fresh and 1 frozen) that was covered under our shared risk program. We were disappointed and discouraged with the news. Our file was transferred to a different doctor at the clinic to see if we wished to continue with another cycle. She reviewed our file and was not very optimistic. She explained that if we were to move forward with another cycle she believed our chances of having a biological child were less than ten percent. Gut punch. She suggested our best chance for success would be to use donor eggs. I simply couldn't understand why my body was betraying me at such a young age. We'd endured a miscarriage, D&C, three retrieval surgeries, three failed cycles, hundreds of shots, suppositories, patches, pills, thousands of dollars spent, loads of anxiety and stress, countless doctor's appointments and still no baby. Now our chances had taken a nosedive. Our hope was continually being dashed with our physical circumstances.

After the donor egg recommendation, I pushed the confusion, hurt, doubt, shame, and frustration down deep. I'd been burying my feelings the entire time and thought I was doing a pretty good job handling things. I'd managed to keep a positive demeanor around family, friends, coworkers, and my students even though many times I felt hopeless, sad, angry, and depressed. Kelley was the only one who truly knew the hell I was walking through because he was right there with me every day supporting me while simultaneously dealing with his own feelings. I've heard everyone has their breaking point and it was while I was looking online at donor egg profiles that I had mine. As I was scrolling the profiles, I filtered through them desperately looking for women who shared several of my physical traits. There were only a few and none that matched completely. Panic rose up like never before because it felt like the dream of being able to dote over my baby and discuss if they got my eyes, hair color, or whatever trait from me was gone. It was too much for me. I felt robbed of the opportunity to use my own eggs and completely overwhelmed with all we'd faced so far. Total hopelessness hit me and I fell out of the chair onto my knees, sobbing inconsolably. Kelley heard me from the other room and came in to hold me until I calmed down. He was an amazing comforter and encourager. Other than the miscarriage, it was my lowest point.

After we talked, I went out to the front porch to watch the sunset and get some fresh air. I remember rehashing the events of our IVF and feeling utterly frustrated and devastated with our situation. It was all consuming. It seemed that every woman my age around me was getting pregnant. *Why not me?* I was surrounded with amazing students every day. *Why couldn't I have a child of my own?* I was struggling with my identity as a woman and as a Christian. *Why couldn't my body do what it was physiologically created to do? Was I praying enough? Believing enough?* (Spoiler alert: there is no "enough"–thank goodness it's not up to our efforts). I felt like a failure and experienced isolation like never before. The hope-despair rollercoaster of infertility treatments was wreaking havoc on my mental health. To add insult to injury, the physical toll of the medication's side effects and financial stresses weighed heavily as well. I also felt so much shame because of the intense grief and emotions I couldn't control, despite all the support from so many. My frustration with God was at an all-time high. Don't get me wrong, I knew I was blessed in so many other ways, however, I couldn't understand why God would withhold one of my most desired dreams–to carry a child and become a mother. It frustrated me in my soul.

As I continued sitting on the porch, I moved my gaze from the sunset to the landscaping right in front of my feet and saw a purple flower. Purple has always been my favorite color, and normally I would have admired the hue or the shape of the petals. However, my state of mind was fragile and the hurt I felt deep down turned into jealousy of that flower. It didn't make sense to me; *even nature could reproduce with ease, so what the heck was wrong with me?* I felt anger and shame. We were working so hard doing everything we could to achieve a pregnancy, *so why wasn't the work ethic I'd known my whole life paying off now?* I felt cheated. I also felt somewhat unstable for being jealous of a flower and questioned my sanity. I'd hit a mental wall in a way I hadn't before. I cried a few more tears and calmed down a bit before I went into the house. After my freak-out session, I felt a wave of comfort come over me. It was like God was giving me even more hope for the future because all of my own hope was gone. I didn't know it at the time, but that small purple flower would be used to challenge and stretch my faith.

A few weeks later I had lunch with friends at an adorable local tearoom. While we were waiting to be seated, I browsed a display case with handmade items for sale. My eyes were drawn to a dainty lace headband with a purple flower attached. The visual of me placing it on a baby girl of my own flashed in my mind and filled me with a split second of excitement and pride. My protective side quickly kicked into high gear and squelched any thought of actually buying it. Thoughts like, *"can you imagine having to get rid of that if you never have a baby? It would hurt way too much"* ran through my head. I continued to browse, but I couldn't deny the moment I'd seen the purple flower at my feet after pouring out my frustrations to God and now the similarity of the purple flower there on that headband. *Was that a coincidence? Probably,* I told myself. I just couldn't do it. I convinced myself that not buying the headband was the safer choice.

I couldn't stop thinking about the purple headband and for over a week it kept coming to my mind. I remember shaming myself about how other women complete whole nurseries in faith while waiting to build their families, and here I was hesitating to buy a little ol' headband. It was strange to me that I didn't have a problem going to doctors' visits or giving myself hundreds of shots, but it felt risky and unsafe to buy a physical reminder of my dreams. I felt the prompting to just buy it and God would do the rest. A sense of relief passed over me as I remembered I didn't need a gigantic faith. All I needed was a little. I've heard a time or two that only a mustard seed-sized faith will do, and so that's what I offered.

I went back and bought the headband with the purple flower. Though small, it was my first tangible, hold-it-in-your-hand step toward releasing my control over our journey and beginning to fully trust God.

We found ourselves at a crossroads in our journey. We'd been told the odds were stacked against us, yet at the same time I began to feel a sense of peace. We'd done everything we could to make our dream of becoming parents happen, yet we had come up empty-handed. Though heartbreaking, in the strangest way it was freeing. I was learning to truly trust God in our loss of perceived control. I'd heard a lot about trusting God and now I was learning firsthand what that actually looked like when there wasn't much hope left. Our dream of being parents hadn't changed, and we would still pursue that, but I also began to feel a peace about how that would happen. Adoption and the use of donor eggs were two options Kelley and I began to discuss. I realized our lives might end up looking differently than we had expected and was beginning to accept that.

During this time, I researched adoption and continued to learn more about both of our diagnoses. Through my research, especially on Kelley's diagnosis, I kept returning to the website of an infertility clinic located in St. Louis that specialized in male factor infertility. My understanding of what I was reading about the clinic and doctor suggested that we may still have a chance. I was also slowly learning to be my own (and Kelley's) advocate rather than giving up because of one clinic's opinion. After discussion and prayer, Kelley and I decided to have a consultation with the reproductive endocrinologist at the St. Louis clinic. We had the 80% of money from the failed IVF cycles, so we decided if the doctor believed there was any hope of success at all, we'd try one last time with my own eggs. My grit wasn't gone yet.

The doctor was an older, short man with white hair that wrapped around his balding head. He had a straight-shooter style of communication and jumped right into discussing our situation. This new doctor had already reviewed our large file sent from the previous clinic and immediately began to share his distaste for the actions taken there. He was protectively indignant, and I could tell he was entirely dedicated to his career in a special way. He did a quick examination of Kelley right there in his personal office. I thought it was a little unorthodox, but I could also tell he was doing this to efficiently save time which I appreciated and admired. It turns out that he began his career as an urologist, so in hindsight, it wasn't strange at all. It was then that he began to apologize for our treatment at the previous clinic. He believed we'd both been either misdiagnosed or mistreated. He didn't believe I had DOV and also said I didn't need the metformin for the PCOS diagnosis–if I even had that condition at all. That was incredible news to hear since I'd already quit taking it due to the extreme stomach pain side effect. He also scoffed at the idea of using donor eggs. He said my ovaries had responded by producing fewer eggs because I'd been prescribed too much follicle-stimulating drugs (Gonal-F). I was stunned! My dad, the farmer, had been right. I had suppressed my intuition, but my gut feelings had also been right. I was relieved and validated simultaneously.

Then he moved to Kelley's file. He explained the previous clinic had performed an inferior method for sperm aspiration. They had done TESE (testicular sperm extraction) using a spring-loaded needle to retrieve Kelley's sperm. He explained this procedure was not only painful but hadn't retrieved the high-quality sperm needed for the highest success rate. MESA (microsurgical epididymal sperm aspiration) was the technique he recommended based on Kelley's condition. This doctor pioneered vasectomy reversal and spoke with a confidence we hadn't heard, so we definitely believed him. He knew we wished to use my eggs for another cycle, if possible, so that's what he immediately began to plan for us. He took out an old school handheld recorder and began to record his notes and a possible IVF protocol for us. I was both amused and impressed at the sight of the recorder and also excited about his certainty. He was so different and it was refreshing. After recording the notes, he gave his final thoughts and said we could relax because we were no longer in the lowest category for success but now the highest. We'd moved from less than ten percent to around a sixty percent success rate. He said with conviction he believed he knew how to help us have a baby.

Our entire situation completely changed in a matter of 30 minutes. We walked out of his office in complete shock and with a strong, renewed hope. We scheduled our fifth IVF cycle with a whole new outlook. It seemed like a dream. Surreal. Our second opinion felt like a life-changing second chance.

As we prepared for the new cycle, I had a growing sense of peace about our future. Of course, we were overjoyed with our new and better chances, but we also knew there was still a large probability of failure. Since experience is the ultimate teacher, I prepared for the uncertainty in ways I hadn't before. I began to practice gratitude and count our blessings more often than focusing on what wasn't there. I also began to make other choices for my mental health. One of those choices, which may ruffle some religious feathers, was to not go to the altar for public prayer at our church before this cycle. We attended a charismatic church at the time that put a lot of emphasis on public prayer for the sick. I'd participated this way during the past four cycles and it had been very emotional for me, especially when we continued to face failure. While I definitely believe in prayer, I realized going to the front for public prayer was placing more emphasis on the outcome and adding more emotional distress and disappointment for me. I'd reached a point where I was okay either way with our outcome, so I decided we'd pray in our seats as well as privately with our family and close friends. Ultimately, God was in control, and I rested in that.

If you take away something from our story, please remember the power of listening to your intuition, a second opinion, and holding onto hope. Our twin girls, Klaire and Kenlee, were born from that fifth IVF cycle at the St. Louis clinic. I was given less follicle stimulating medication (Follistim instead of Gonal-f) and MESA was performed for Kelley. Two other embryos were then frozen from the cycle and transferred five years later in our sixth and final cycle. A third daughter, Korinne, was born from the frozen cycle. We had no other embryos left and were blessed with three healthy, beautiful daughters. All three girls were born in the month of November, which was the same month I'd suffered the miscarriage. It was beauty for ashes beyond what we had prayed for. It was a true Ephesians 3:20 story: "immeasurably more than all we ask or imagine, according to His power that is at work within us." All three girls have worn the purple flower headband I bought as an offering of faith. I had an imperfect faith including questions and frustrations, yet it didn't disqualify me from God's blessings.

The details couldn't have been more perfect. It blows my mind that we were blessed with three walking, talking miracles and we credit God and the incredibly talented IVF team. Our girls were 100% worth the battle and now serve as human reminders of God's sovereignty, provision, and blessings. This time in our lives stretched our limits physically, emotionally, and spiritually. It was the most difficult time in my life, but hopefully the following mental health lessons I learned might help you if you are struggling with fertility issues.

Dealing with infertility is grief. Try to recognize and accept your feelings of grief, anger, and frustration rather than deny them or feel shame because of them. They're normal. Infertility does not define you. Be gentle with yourself and your husband and support each other. Sharing reminds you that you're not alone, even when it feels like it; so find support with an individual or group of people going through a similar situation. Practice daily prayer and gratitude and attempt to find joy in the present. Try to limit time on social media and increase your movement and time spent outside. Infertility can be all consuming, so remind yourself that your current circumstances are not your final destination. Much like our story is only one chapter in this book, your infertility battle will only be one chapter in your life. I promise.

As wonderful as our story turned out, I know not all infertility experiences end this way. Just because your story doesn't look like ours doesn't mean you won't end up with your own happy ending, whatever that looks like. God doesn't always answer in the same way for all couples dealing with infertility. Our journey taught us to hang onto hope as we do our best to trust God. It is my prayer that our story can encourage you to do the same in your unique situation. Parts of the process will be messy and that's okay. Our big emotions are never too big for God. I also hope you have your own purple flower moment when you can take a deep breath and begin to rest in the unknowns of the future and trust that God knows your path, so you don't always have to. This is easier said than done, but it is truly a life-changing gift. Finally, I pray one day you'll be able to look back on your infertility journey only as a memory and realize you've gained some valuable lessons and amazing miracles of your own. I'm cheering you on.

REFERENCES

Brown, B,. (2012, March). *Listening to Shame* [Video]. TED Conferences. https://www.ted.com/talks/brene_brown_listening_to_shame?language=en

CHAPTER NINE

JANELY'S STORY
JOY, HOPE, & PERSEVERANCE IN PAIN
By Shawna Landázuri

This story really begins deep in the jungle of Ecuador. A frightened and confused Grandmother sought help for her granddaughter who was very ill. The hospital, seeing that the situation was dire and this baby was in need of extensive medical help, called a local orphanage known for taking on hard and even terminal cases. When the founder of Casa de Fe (translated House of Faith) heard the request, she said "yes" knowing her board would not be thrilled with the decision. Saying "yes" and taking on this baby's care meant many medical bills once again.

The granddaughter in this story is Janely, my daughter. Janely's (pronounced Juh-nell-ee) life is a story of great suffering, heartache, and trauma. However, there is also perseverance, tremendous hope, and profound beauty. But I might be a little biased. God's handiwork is woven through her story and our story, even in the pain. You see, Janely had sustained significant brain damage in her mother's womb. Janely's biological mother tried to end Janely's life by ingesting a poisonous leaf that was known to cause an abortion, but Janely lived. When she was five months old, Janely's mother tragically ended her life with a poisonous leaf and soon after, her grandmother handed over the baby's care to Casa de Fe.

Janely was taken to a private hospital in Quito with a charity wing, which meant services were more affordable. In Ecuador the majority of the population seek care at the public hospitals where the demand is very high and the quality of care is often very poor. Moving her to the private hospital likely saved Janely's life. The doctors discovered that Janely had a parasitic infection that had gone untreated and had caused significant brain trauma and damage. Janely was diagnosed with many things but primarily congenital toxoplasmosis (the parasitic infection), hydrocephalus, and meningitis, along with blindness, epilepsy, and profound developmental delay.

Over the next few months, the orphanage sent missionaries to stay with Janely. She underwent four surgeries to place, and then replace, shunts in her brain to drain the cerebrospinal fluid and attempt to lower the pressure in her brain. The hydrocephalus caused the high pressure and further brain damage. Janely miraculously survived each surgery as well as a life-threatening infection.

In 2010, my future husband Juan Manuel and I crossed paths and he left a great impression on me as a man dedicated to and passionate for the Lord. We met at a life group, in California where I was living at the time, when he attended with his brother and then soon returned to his home in Ecuador. Three years later the Holy Spirit spoke to my sister-in-law and she was faithful to initiate a second connection between the two of us. We had a beautiful and fairly quick romance that started with a friendship that led to courting and then marriage in August of 2013 in Ecuador. Every step of the way God gave us both peace and made details come together as only He could to show us this was His plan. My move to Ecuador and the start of our lives together really showed us both the way God was truly involved in every detail of our lives and desired healing and redemption for each of us. We were both also excited to learn, during our engagement, that we each desired to adopt! We developed a plan to have biological children first and adopt in the middle age-wise hoping that child would feel more a part of the family. Little did we know God was very much in that dream of adoption and He was about to scrap our plan for His own crazy, beautiful plan!

Eight months into our marriage we heard about Janely one Sunday at church. We liked to sit in the front row to eliminate distractions from the message and worship. When our pastor began describing a baby who needed help, my eyes welled up with tears as he mentioned that she had Hydrocephalus. The announcement was asking for a couple to care for this baby until she could "recover" and go back to her grandmother in the jungle. Tears welled up in my eyes as I remembered another infant with Hydrocephalus I had helped to care for at the public hospital as part of the volunteer mission work I was doing.

I remembered our conversation about having our own children and then adopting. I also knew we had agreed we wouldn't talk about starting our family until we had been married for one year. Knowing it was too early, I decided not to say a word about this opportunity. Following the service, our pastor approached us and said that he had noticed our eyes when he announced the baby needing help, and wanted to know if we would be willing to pray about this opportunity. You don't really tell your pastor "no" when he asks you to pray so we said "yes, of course!" Later that night I prayed and asked God that if He wanted this for us, would He please "do the work in my husband's heart." I knew that sometimes these situations could turn into adoption and wanted to know without a shadow of a doubt that I had no part whatsoever in trying to influence the situation, despite how badly I wanted to say yes. After that prayer, life went on as usual for a few weeks with no mention at all of the baby.

One Saturday we were watching a sermon online as we always did, but this day Juan Ma' (short for Juan Manuel) paused it mid-sermon. He explained how he felt the Lord was prompting us to live with open hands with all the blessings we had and maybe that meant opening our home to this baby. He wanted to know what I thought. Right then my heart began beating faster with excitement. We talked, prayed, and agreed to move forward. Even though we lived in a tiny one-bedroom apartment and were on a small, missionary budget, we were so in love, felt our cup was overflowing with God's blessings, and wanted to help others. Let it be known, I did not hear anything from the online sermon that Juan Ma' had that day, which was just evidence to me that God did indeed "do the work" in my husband's heart just as I had asked.

In the next two months we had an honest conversation with one of the staff at the orphanage that was responsible for making the decision where to place Janely. Two other couples were also interested. We were invited to meet Janely and pray for her in the hospital, which we did. The time with her was fairly uneventful so we waited. I remember thinking, *this is surreal; surely this kind of thing won't happen to me.* A few weeks later we learned we had been selected to take care of Janely simply because her pediatrician liked the idea of a couple with no other children due to the danger of germs and her weakened immune system. There were several delays in her discharge as another shunt surgery was needed and recovery took longer than planned. It continued to feel as though it would never actually happen until I got the call. On May 31, 2014, I went to stay with Janely in the hospital after her fourth brain surgery and from that moment on, she did not leave our sight. Janely was three days short of nine months old.

The first day with Janely felt surreal and I worked hard with every silly sound I knew to get a reaction from her but just got flattened affect and glazed-over eyes. I prayed that day for God to create a connection between Janely and me so I could love her the best way possible. It has always been hard to admit that there was not an immediate connection, but I love to share how God answers prayers. Shortly after I prayed that prayer, I put Janely in my lap, tubes and all, and after a few moments she laid her head on my chest and fell asleep. That did it! The love and connection was practically instantaneous!

The following months were full of doctor's appointments and falling deeper in love with Janely's caramel colored skin and black eyes we affectionately called her "black pearls." After two weeks with us Janely's shunt was blocked again requiring yet another surgery. Then two and a half months later she had her sixth shunt replacement surgery. Asking a lot of questions is not well received in the Ecuadorian culture from a patient to a doctor, but I had to advocate for Janely and try to understand why things were not improving. The message became very clear whether I was talking with her neurosurgeon, neurologist, or pediatrician—Janely would never "recover" but would always need to live close to a neurosurgery team that could act quickly in an emergency. Through this time God's goodness was evident in many ways including His provision of an English-speaking Pediatrician who was an angel to our family as my Spanish was so limited.

Each day I would share with Juan Ma' what I had learned about the severity of Janely's condition, as he was working during the day to support us and could not be there for all the many, many doctor's appointments and therapy visits. I realized her need for care was too high for her to live with her grandmother in the jungle. Their family had no transportation of their own and it was two bus rides and about eight hours away to the closest neurosurgery team in Quito. This was not including the therapy we attended several times a week to see if Janely could learn to hold her head up or move her hands or body on her own. I remember how much I struggled in this season with not being able to call myself her Mom as I fell deeper in love with her. I couldn't imagine not having her in my life and then wondered if she would be well cared for. As a recovering high-performer and perfectionist, I also struggled a lot with the pressure of helping her "recover" when we took on her care. There was lots of wrestling with God and hard conversations with my husband about adopting her when we saw her medical bills coming in. We had no financial solvency but were actually praying and waiting for donations from our supporters to come in month to month. Looking back now it is so reassuring to see God had a plan; we just weren't privy to it yet, and it was a beautiful plan! I also see how God used Janely to teach me to trust Him in my weakness and despite my faults. We can glorify His name all the more when there is a victory knowing it was His work and not my own just as Paul describes in 2 Corinthians 12:9, "Each time he said, 'My grace is all you need. My power works best in weakness.' So now I am glad to boast about my weaknesses, so that the power of Christ can work through me."

My husband said, "Janely is the best missionary I've ever known!" Let me explain. Many Ecuadorians saw me—light skin, light eyes, and obviously Caucasian—and saw Janely and asked questions. This gave me countless opportunities to answer their questions that often lead to "why?" They wanted to know why we would adopt a child because adoption is often looked down on in Ecuadorian culture (though we see that slowly changing). Therefore, to adopt a child with a different ethnicity and medical and special needs was very shocking. We loved getting to share how Jesus had adopted us and shown us the most life-changing love we had ever known; it was a great, great privilege to adopt and get a tiny glimpse of what He has done for us. To be honest, Janely was also completely adorable and so very easy to love!

This also might be a good time to mention that Janely's unresponsiveness had begun to change shortly after bringing her home. I grew up singing, and it was always a form of therapy for me and simply something I loved to do. Every day at home we sang worship songs and I tried to get Janely to make sounds. Little by little she responded with a sound, grunt, or coo of some sort. I will never forget exactly where she was laying in her crib that day, in a violet-colored onesie, when she gave me a sweet little smirk while I was singing to her. Worship and song became Janely's most favorite thing in the world and for a woman who needs to be singing, it was clear we were a perfect fit!

On our first wedding anniversary, we realized it was time to make a final decision on whether to pursue Janely's adoption. We were back and forth but due to financial concerns we were worried we wouldn't be able to adequately take care of her. That night we prayed again and then agreed to put all the cards on the table. We talked about how looking at her significant level of disability and medical needs we may not be able to manage having biological children as well and could we be okay with that? I fell even deeper in love with my husband through this process watching him try to help our family make a good decision as well as seeing his love for Janely. We both agreed that while we would love to have a child that looked like both of us, we don't "need" that and were willing to give that up if that is what it would take to make Janely ours. We did not really know or understand fully at that point all we were saying "yes" to and "no" to. But I know that God gave us His heart for Janely so that we would have the desire and strength to want to make that sacrifice. I also believe that there are many things He does not allow us to fully know because we would run the other way. But when that hard day or season comes, He will walk with us and carry us through!

Juan Ma' and I came to the conclusion in August 2014, shortly before her first birthday, that we could not fathom letting her go; we committed to her adoption. This began a process that lasted a little over three years. All this time was spent running around the city for documents, translations, lawyers' visits, interviews, multiple home studies, an extensive psychiatric evaluation, all with Janely right next to me in a cab. Doctor's visits continued along with therapy and hospitalizations for many types of exams, respiratory problems, seizures, more shunt surgeries, and a significant hip displacement requiring two surgeries. Janely's list of conditions and complexity of care grew and the diagnosis of quadriplegia and intractable epilepsy (meaning it is not controlled with two or more medications) were added along with others.

Our hope was to get Janely to the United States as soon as possible for better medical care, access to more medications for her seizures, and more advanced therapy to help her possibly learn to hold up her head. During this time we were denied a special type of Visa that would help us get Janely to the US faster. I struggled to understand why God would not grant us this request when Janely's need was so great and the doctors in Ecuador seemed to be running out of options. I remember God putting it on my heart to look up as many scriptures as I could find about waiting. I was pleasantly surprised and definitely encouraged to keep waiting after reading how God blesses those who wait. As Isaiah 30:18 says, "Therefore the Lord waits to be gracious to you, and therefore He exalts Himself to show mercy to you. For the Lord is a God of justice; blessed are all those who wait for Him."

As we lived life with our baby girl, we learned how to celebrate every little victory. Holding her head up a few seconds longer while on her tummy was huge and we erupted into cheering and screaming each time. I remember how excited we were the first time Janely was able to touch her little fist (her hands were always clenched due to the Cerebral Palsy) to my husband's face, or when I noticed her trying to sing with me by trying to match the key. When you spend every day doing exercises and stretches taught to you by physical, occupational and/or speech therapists, every small victory feels enormous and exciting. We all worked very hard. The learning curve was huge for me as a first time mom learning Spanish. Juan Ma' and I were so excited if we thought up a new idea that would help her or find something that she enjoyed. You see, when your child cannot see, touch, or move when or where she wants, finding a toy that she enjoys with your help was a big challenge; it taught us how to brainstorm, persevere, and again celebrate regularly!

On January 9th, 2017, Janely's adoption was approved! We enjoyed choosing her middle name "Hope" to demonstrate how God had plucked her out of the jungle and given her a different and hopeful story! She had endured a significant emergency hospitalization for one month in 2016 when we were minutes away from losing her, so when we celebrated, it was for far more than her adoption. We were finally able to start making concrete plans to move to the United States and let Janely meet the rest of her family. As I look back over the journey of adoption, I am so grateful we were able to foster Janely until the process was complete so that we had those years to love and take care of her. We also saw perhaps why God did not allow the first Visa to be approved. International adoption costs are significantly higher than a local adoption in Ecuador and we needed finances for our move and starting from scratch with only six bags of belongings. He also gave us a very special group of people in our local church that helped us through the journey and loved Janely. I cannot imagine completely understanding all the reasons why God did what He did but time has given me perspective to see His plan was beautiful. I know I truly would not have wanted it any other way. Perhaps some of His biggest work was teaching me to wait on Him and trust Him more.

After we moved to the US, there were many obstacles we did not foresee about her paperwork and medical coverage that God took care of in His time. During seasons of financial hardship, God never failed to come through, even when it was down to the wire. Janely's health also did not magically improve as I hadn't realized I had been hoping. I began building her team of specialists, doctors, and therapists quickly. Janely hit a new season of worsened seizures for ten months and, in the middle of that, became very ill with a respiratory virus that, in conjunction with seizures, brought us to the second time we almost lost her this side of heaven.

Over the years, Janely's health, diagnoses, and level of care progressively became more and more complex. She was diagnosed with neuromuscular scoliosis, developed severe reflux and aspiration issues (when fluid or secretions go into the lungs instead of stomach), and her muscles grew tighter from the effect of Cerebral Palsy. This was all despite the rigid schedule of therapy and stretching and the transition to a feeding tube in 2016. However, even through the many battles she fought, God continued to give us enormous victories! Janely's eyesight improved enough to see movement and light. This ultimately led to a form of communication, such as looking at an adapted card made for her type of vision loss to show us what color she wanted her wheelchair to be or which toy she wanted to play with. I smile as I write this remembering how exciting it was to know which color she wanted for her wheelchair!

Janely also began taking steps in her gait trainer after over a year of hard work. A gait trainer is like a walker attached to her body that has a seat to give her body and trunk support along with elbow pads for leaning forward. Singing at the top of our lungs while she was in her gait trainer was our favorite activity. She was excited and wanted to be close to our faces when we sang so she would move her little legs and come after us. After years and years of many types of therapy, this was nothing short of miraculous when you consider the very poor prognosis we had been given.

Life went on with many procedures and visits to approximately thirteen doctors and specialists, not including second opinions or additional one-time visits with sub-specialists within an area of medical specialty. Janely had eleven surgeries and more hospital stays and visits to the emergency room than I could count. She received physical, speech, occupational, and vision therapy from therapists in outpatient clinics as well as from her school. She even rode a horse with three people helping her for four and a half years at a therapy clinic we called our second home. In His compassion, God also sent many nurses and caregivers into our lives to help us in our home and in some cases, they became like family to us and gave us the beautiful gift of their friendship.

On July 11, 2023, Janely left her physical body behind to join Jesus in heaven. Her complex medical issues had progressively worsened and went beyond what her physical body could handle despite the medical interventions. We miss our daughter terribly, yet we truly feel that being her parents was the greatest privilege of our lives! You see, Janely was easy to please and we saw her traverse many hardships and physical pain but with a small kiss or a song, she emanated joy! As we cared for her, we also learned to persevere through the greatest pains of our lives. I faced many health issues and chronic sleep deprivation over the years that was debilitating at times. However, my husband and I both learned how to keep going when we did not know how we physically could and we concluded it was God's supernatural work in us. I learned how to worship God with song through excruciating seasons of pain.

Our hearts were broken over and over again during the nine and a half years we were blessed to be Janely's parents. I struggled often with why God allowed her to suffer so much when she was innocent and He has the power to heal her. While I do not have the full answer, God patiently and lovingly showed me that despite her great suffering, He will make it all beautiful in His time. I was blessed in Janely's life to see some of the ways He used her and her story to show others His radical love. Often strangers simply approached me and shared what they saw as we lived a normal day in our very different lives. I was also reminded during Janely's life on earth and afterwards that the best gift God can give anyone is Himself! God so clearly used Janely's life to give us more of Him. Our lives were so consumed with caregiving that it was often hard to leave the house. Every scenario required so much planning, equipment, and special spaces to change her diaper or catheterize her that we left our home less and less. We also wanted to protect her from germs and viruses knowing that they would harm her ten times worse than someone with a normal immune system. Our isolated homebound life forced us to turn to God even more, humble ourselves to receive help, and spend time worshiping Him and watching Janely get super excited when we did!

The way God shaped our family is very special to us but never looked like we imagined. By turning to God and praying for His help and guidance, we can say with total confidence that God called us to be Janely's parents and that was monumental for us. More times than I could count, when we were discouraged, we would look back to the beginning of our story and remind ourselves that God called us to this life. We were on a kingdom mission every single day! When I was able to see every detail of Janely's care as not only trying to love my daughter well but as a kingdom mission, it helped me trust that He would work it out in a beautiful way! I remember after I had to leave the majority of the traditional mission work in ministries in Ecuador to take care of Janely, I would often struggle with day-to-day life. Changing diapers was an occurrence every single day for nine and half years and was often very messy, very time consuming and, as she grew older, a physically challenging task. I remember God teaching me that when I gently wiped her bottom or slid off her poop-filled pants with extra care, I was loving His little girl and that gave Him pleasure. I pictured God smiling on both of us and when I remembered that I was able to enjoy taking care of Janely not only as a mom in love with her little girl, but also to feel delight in my heavenly Father delighting in me!

There are more details of our story with Janely than I can cover here. I also cannot begin to recount God's faithfulness in one chapter because there were so many small and big ways God came through for us. I don't have perfect answers to my questions or why Janely's life involved so much suffering and ended too soon. What I can attest to is that though my fears and doubts have gotten the best of me at times over the years, God has always been there with us. He put a wonderful community around us in some seasons and in others we struggled and felt very alone. Again, I can see how He drew us in deeper to His heart and taught us how to endure suffering and still worship Him. I see how God chose a husband for me that would be a "battle buddy" for me by my side in the trenches of Janely's care far beyond what I ever thought any man would be willing to do. It all comes back to God's loving attention to every detail of our lives. He chose the three of us for each other whether it was being a part of each other's healing or being a part of His refining work in our lives. Motherhood was my greatest privilege and joy (even with all the pain) and I trust I will see more and more of God's hand in Janely's life and our story as time goes on. Until we see her again, we are imagining her totally healed and free to dance and sing with Jesus "in fullness of joy" from Psalms 16:11, "You make known to me the path of life; in your presence there is fullness of joy; at your right hand are pleasures forevermore."

CHAPTER TEN

OUR PLANS VS. GOD'S PLANS

By Lindsey Racz

In 2019, after 18 years of being a follower of Christ, I read the entire Bible completely and chronologically for the first time. I had been reading scripture for many years in smaller chunks, usually one chapter at a time, but somehow the task of reading it from start to finish had felt overwhelming. Finally, when my faith was mature, I decided it was time. A beautiful, cohesive, and overarching understanding of God's heart was the gift I received from reading His word this way.

In Genesis we see God become the Father to humankind. He is thrilled and plans to have us live out our days in the beautiful garden He's created–the perfect place for His new children to thrive! One problem. He gives His new creation free will. He does this because of one word. LOVE. God, in His infinite wisdom, wants to love and be loved freely by His babies! Forced love wouldn't really be love at all.

Now we see the enemy of God's children enter the story. Serpent evil. One of the biggest problems we face as we try to love God and live out His plans for our lives is that there's another power at work in this world. The bible calls Satan "the prince of this world" and "the father of lies." It's important for us to recognize that we have a very real enemy who hates God and is in open rebellion against Him and

His beloved creation. Satan wants to convince us that God doesn't have our best interest in mind and that He's probably withholding good things from us. When we start believing those lies, we are right where our enemy wants us to be; separated from God.

It is easy for us in our human condition to listen to Satan. We doubt our good Father. We bite the apple. Broken-hearted, Father must protect us from ourselves. Now we have the knowledge of both good and evil. Oh, how ignorance had been bliss.

The rest of the story reads like this: God continues to pursue His children who continue to go their own way. He makes a plan to rescue us. A big, epic, never-been-tried-before plan. He's God, so He knows the plan will work. It's the only way. Because we had willfully given up our freedom, He sends His heavenly Son to trade places. To trade His freedom for our bondage. Darkest night. Blood drenched wood. Stench of death. Serpent evil celebrates.

But only for three days.

God has a plan involving an empty tomb and eternal life not just for His heavenly Son, but also for all of His children. A new plan. A new dream.

It's glorious. Satan screeches. He's been defeated and he knows it. God, the ultimate Father, has found a way to care for and be with His babies forever. They still have free will, thus there is only one choice that matters. They have to want to be with Him too. Forever. And then, even though their human body will wear out, their spirit will live on. Forever. In God's new garden, a place called Heaven.

The end of the Bible tells us that He's coming back for those of us who have died and those of us who are still alive. He's coming back for those of us who have trusted in Him as our only hope. And we will be knit not only spiritually, but also physically, into the biggest, best family in the entire world. God's family. I can't imagine a better plan or a better end to the story. I can't imagine a better family for you, for me . . . for all of us.

But before we get there, there are valleys to cross, hills to climb, and yes, tears to cry. There are lessons we must learn to help us develop into all He has for us. Contrary as it seems, the valleys aren't cruel, but kind. We must be ready for our heavenly realities, and as it turns out, valleys are great training grounds.

When I sat down to draft the last chapter of this book, I had just finished reading through each author's story. Although we did not collaborate on progression of themes to write our stories, each chapter reads like this: an idea of how our life will unfold, reality not matching that idea, a mad attempt to control our outcomes, a desperate and often unwanted surrender, a bend in the road, the path looking different, the eventual surrender of our dream, grief, and then, a new dream. A new plan.

Our stories–and your story–are about letting go of all we thought we should have. In exchange, we can grab hold of what God has for us. And He is a God of miracles. There are parts of our stories we still don't understand and won't pretend to, and yet we are beginning to see, bit by bit, that these stories are indeed *the* plan. There are riches in these new stories that wouldn't have been found had our lives matched the perfect scripts we had constructed for ourselves.

Oh yes, we wrestled with God and still do. As we wrestle, God is busy writing lessons, truths, and treasures into our hearts that can only become concrete through struggle. He has a good plan even when His "good" doesn't seem to align with our understanding of good.

In the book of Genesis, we learn the story of Joseph. It's one of my favorites. If you've never read it, check out Genesis chapters 37–50. In my summation, Joseph starts off as a bit of an arrogant teenager. He's the baby of the family and his parents' favorite child. He also has the gift of prophetic dreams but hasn't yet figured out how to share these dreams tactfully. His older brothers resent him and actually sell him into slavery, telling their parents that Joseph has been killed. His father mourns. His brothers secretly cheer; they've gotten rid of their smug brother.

Little do the people in this story know that God is actually writing a much bigger story behind the scenes. You see, God has incredible plans for Joseph. He wants to make him into a prince and ultimately use him to save many peoples' lives. But Joseph is nowhere near ready for this big calling on his life. He needs character development. So, what does God do? He allows Joseph to experience hardship.

Notice that I am choosing the word "allows" over the word "causes" intentionally here. There is a complex interplay between what is caused by the enemy and what God allows to touch our lives that I am not sure we will be able to understand on this side of heaven. Romans 8:28 says "And we know that in all things God works for the good of those who love him, who have been called according to his purpose." The enemy can cause bad things and God can use those things for His purposes.

Difficult things happen to Joseph. He is sold into slavery. He faces false accusations against his character. He becomes a prisoner for years. He's beaten. His hardships are innumerable. But in the end, Joseph's character is developed through these hardships. He never stops seeking the Lord. Because of this, he is eventually assigned as Pharaoh's personal advisor and becomes a high-ranking official in the Egyptian court. He forgives his brothers, models great compassion, and ultimately, saves an entire civilization from famine. In Genesis 50:20, Joseph's famous line summarizes his whole story as he speaks directly to his brothers, "You intended to harm me, but God intended it for good to accomplish what is now being done, the saving of many lives."

Could it be that hardship is actually a blessing in disguise, as was the case for Joseph? It wouldn't seem that hard things could actually be good, but there's this peculiar pattern in Scripture that seems to be on repeat. We are told that in the Kingdom of Heaven, for example, the first shall be last and the last shall be first (Matthew 20:16). We are told that those who humble themselves will be exalted, and those who exalt themselves will be humbled (Matthew 23:12). "Blessed are those who mourn." (Matthew 5:4) Really? Mourning is a blessing? Have you ever deeply mourned someone or something? It sure doesn't *feel* like a blessing. And yet scripture tells us the person who is mourning is blessed. What if in our very finite minds and with our human emotions, we actually aren't sure what's good for us in the big picture? What if we don't know what we need and we misunderstand the concept of good altogether?

To see this in my everyday life, I need to look no further than parenting. My four-year-old gets a timeout and a stern talking to, and is abruptly removed from his tricycle, after he decides to ride on the road. My five-year-old cries on her way to the school co-op every day, "I don't want to go to school!" My fourteen-year-old huffs, "Why can't I just have social media? Mom, you're so overprotective!" Our eighteen-year-old calls from California excited about a cool credit card offer he got. We squash his excitement with financial advice. And there we have it, four times over, our interactions with our kids feel negative to each of them. How on earth could we want good for them?

But protecting a toddler from riding in the road, giving a very shy six-year-old a safe place to practice social skills, helping a new teen avoid online dangers, and advising a young adult to run from debt are all acts of love. These acts are for their good, even if they aren't able to see that at this time.

Our sight is limited too. We can't see our Father's love for us as we walk through hardship, are removed from a path of danger, get the "no" answer, or learn a difficult lesson. What if we looked beyond our human capacity to understand and chose faith? Faith is being "sure of what we hope for and certain of what we cannot see." (Hebrews 11:1). I hope God is ultimately, deeply, and immeasurably good, so I'm choosing to be sure of this. I trust He has good lined up for my future. I hope that each hard thing that has crossed my path has been painstakingly allowed by a heavenly Father who knew it was exactly what I needed to learn in order to become all that He has for me.

So, what can we do as we wait for God to show us goodness while facing bad news? I want to introduce you to a concept from an incredible book called *Thriving Despite a Difficult Marriage*, brilliantly authored by marriage therapists—brothers and Christian Psychologists—Dr. Michael Misja and Dr. Chuck Misja.

Drs. Michael and Chuck Misja introduce three worldviews that are common, especially in Christian circles in the West, which can apply not only in marital situations but also throughout life in general. The first is Happily Ever After. Happily Ever After is the belief that if we have enough faith, we work and pray hard enough, and we follow the right steps, all will turn out as we hope. It's the fairy tale ending. The only problem with Happily Ever After, of course, is that it's not a biblical model, at least not on this side of eternity. Jesus himself tells us that "in this world we will have trouble," but he continues with this line of hope, "Take heart, I have overcome the world." (John 16:33b).

Noble Suffering is the next common worldview. Noble Suffering aligns with the fact that there is suffering in this world. Noble Suffering says we can do nothing about this suffering but bravely endure it and pray for strength. Noble suffering could almost be accurate, except for the fact that it puts us in a victim role. God never intended for us to be powerless victims. His word says that although we may suffer, He's come to give us "abundant life". (John 10:10).

The last and most hope-inducing worldview introduced by Dr. Chuck and Dr. Michael is Thriving Despite. Thriving Despite does not find peace in the denial of life's challenges, such as Happily Ever After does. Thriving Despite does not leave us powerlessly trapped in a broken life. Thriving Despite says that even when hard, unplanned things come our way, we can, in fact, thrive! We do this by coming to terms with and fully grieving our disappointments, releasing attempts to try to control outcomes, and looking for good in any areas of life we can find. We will all have our own wilderness to walk through. Thriving Despite says that even when pain is part of our story, there's still room in our hands and hearts to hold and make beauty. It's a beautiful hope. (Misja & Misja 2009).

Katherine Wolf is one of my favorite authors in the whole world. Her story can be read by visiting her website, HopeHeals.com. A quick overview (that leaves out so many of the important details) is that Katherine's life plans and dreams were completely derailed, she fought for her life, she fought for joy, and eventually through years of struggle, she figured out how to access both life and joy in the face of dying dreams.

You will see one of her powerful life mottos right on the landing page of her website: "We're disrupting the myth that joy can only be found in a pain free life." (Wolf, 2020). You will want to pick up both of her books. Start with *Hope Heals* and then read *Suffer Strong*. Thank me later.

I've heard Katherine speak twice. Both times were life-changing experiences for me. Katherine will tell you that there is a lot we can lose in this life, but there are several things we can never lose: things that lead to a life of brilliant hope and joy. We can lose homes, jobs, our health, and even loved ones. We can lose dreams. But those things which cannot be stolen? Read this list slowly:

1. Peace of conscience
2. Joy of the Holy Spirit
3. Fruition of God's presence in this life
4. Assurance of God's faith in the next life

Take a moment to reread and inhale those truths.

Dearest reader, I don't know what dream you might have to let go of. I don't know what dream is possibly being pried away from you right now. I don't know where you stand with God or even who you believe Him to be. I know you may be seeking answers, so I want to gently say this: don't stop. Dig into this hard season because there are treasures hidden in the darkness for you (Isaiah 45:3).

As you try to shape your family and your life, I implore you to ask new questions. Yes, you can ask God directly, "Why am I struggling with infertility? Why did the adoption fall through again? Why is my child sick? Why did you take my child away?" These are very valid questions. But don't stop there. Begin a new string of questions, "Who is God, really? What does He have for me in this valley? What does God's goodness mean for me, personally?"

You want a family, and we, the storytellers of these pages, deeply understand this aching desire. We have each become intimately familiar with the surrender of our plans and the freedom that, against all odds, surrender brings. When you let go of your dream, it will feel scary. But this very act makes room for a new dream. A God-sized dream. This new dream may look very close to your original dream, or it may be so unrecognizable that it doesn't even feel like your life. What if that's okay? What if your life could look completely different from how you planned and that could actually be good? Not in a good-that-feels-good sort of way, but in an upside-down-Kingdom-good sort of way? What if you could thrive while not receiving the plan you had in mind? I believe you can. And I only know this because I've lived it. Those of us who walk these paths will know a deeper kind of good, we'll know a life of richer understanding and deeper compassion.

As we come to the end of this book, you have steps ahead of you. Your next step may involve getting off social media because seeing others celebrate new babies is too painful right now. Your next step may look like wrestling with God through prayers at three in the morning and begging Him to show you His good plan for your life. Your next step might be fighting for joy on your knees in prayer. It might be committing to read through God's word completely and chronologically for the first time, or the first time in a long time.

If your next step is to truly lean into Jesus Christ, there is one promise I can make to you: your arms will not remain empty. They cannot. His tomb was empty so that your life would not be. His promises are never empty because He is a God of fullness. Your life, your dreams, your well-being, all mean more to Him than this book could ever come close to conveying. Dear sister, dear reader, dear mom-in-waiting, rest assured that something is being birthed in you at this very moment.

The plotline of your life is big, God is even bigger, and your story is being written right now. "May the God of hope fill you with all joy and peace as you trust in Him, so that you may overflow with hope by the power of the Holy Spirit" (Romans 15:13).

REFERENCES

Kubler-Ross, E., & Kessler, D, (2014) *On Grief and Grieving: Finding the Meaning of Grief through the Five Stages of Loss*. New York: Simon & Schuster.

Misja, M., & Misja, C. (2009).*Thriving despite a difficult marriage*. Colorado Springs: NavPress

Wolf, K., (2020). Hope Heals. https://hopeheals.com/

ACKNOWLEDGMENTS

To birth moms everywhere—you chose life, and your brave choice filled empty houses. We see you. Thank you for your courageous sacrifice.

To my husband Matt who supported me through meltdowns when I worried I would not be able to bring this book to fruition. Indeed, you reminded me this was and is God's project and it was never up to me to begin with. Thank you, my loving and faithful best friend.

To my very first miracle babe, Brooke. I'm sorry I had to learn how to be a mom on you! You've been gracious to me. Your spunky spirit always reminds me that God is in the details. You are so very on purpose, my dear.

To our first-round editors, Elizabeth and Ann-Marie, at Best Words Copy. Thank you for making our rough edges as smooth as Canadian butter! Your investment in us is priceless. To Terah Hensley who took a risk on editing a big project. Your countless hours led to one cohesive knitting of God's beautiful grace right here in these very pages. I am in awe of your gifts and grateful to call you cousin and friend. Here's to honoring our dads!

To Karen, Melissa, Jennifer, Shawna, Laura, Terah, Kristina, and Kelsey. An email came out of the blue asking you to share your heart with the public on the pages of a God-sized project! Some of you had never even met me, a few of you barely knew me, and those of you who did know me—well, your risk was biggest of all! Thank you for your *yes*. May the God of hope multiply your work, dreams, and deepest longings through the sharing of your testimony.

Thank you to our incredibly faithful donors: Hilkiah Cortez, Karen Hester, Brandi O'Reilly, Joanne Ridderbos, Jami Bryan, Mellissa Frietchen, Emily Kimbrough, Denise Morgan, Jacque Jackson, Tal Kroll, Ronda

Thomas, Stacy Johannsen, Lauren Short, Miranda Johnston, Bengie K Gray, Traci Garrison, Pamela S Stafford, Mary Eckrich, Lauren Franke, Emily Landis, Denise Meyer, Kylie McMahon, Carlie and Katie Fischer, Serina Mccrea, Sarah Wilson, Laura Picker, Beth Burch, Corbin Caruthers, Christy Hannegan, Susan Wiggs, Darryl Lace, Michael and Ruth Campbell, Diana Fortner, Lacey Kinzer, Jeanne Rich, Menditto David, Dana Burnich, Lindsay Fortson, Kendra Ray, Barbara Herrmann, Artiona Mehmetaj, Stephanie Soto, Diane Rau, Ceara Barmeier, Kathryn Hampton, Caitlin Kissee and Lindsay Puddy. We asked for help with publishing costs and you SHOWED UP! Without your support this book would not be in the hands of those who desperately need to know they aren't alone.

To Lauren Short, for lending your classy design-eye when my husband and I had too many cover options to keep straight. What a gorgeous book we have, thanks to you!

To my mom. As I parent, age, learn, and go through heartaches, I see more clearly all that you walked through to raise Olivia and me. Thank you for reading to me and helping me make books when I was little. I'll be fortunate to become half the mom you were and still are.

ABOUT THE AUTHOR

Lindsey Racz is a follower of Jesus, a wife, and a mom to four miracle babes. She is a Licensed Professional Counselor, founder, and co-owner of the women's mental health clinic, Truth and Counsel, LLC. With over a decade of therapy practice, her areas of specialty include a certification in Cognitive Behavioral Therapy, and a certification in Brain Health Coaching. She holds both bachelor's and master's degrees in Psychology.

Lindsey's desire is to be a light for Christ in all she does; she enjoys using her testimony to help minister to women. She and her family reside in Springfield, Missouri where you will find them outside in the sunshine anytime it's available.

Made in the USA
Columbia, SC
18 December 2024

49808243R00086